Clinical Dental Hygiene

Clinical Dental Hygiene

A handbook for the dental team

T. F. Walsh, DDS, MSc., BDS, FDSRCS(Eng)
*Senior Lecturer and Consultant in Restorative
Dentistry, University of Sheffield, UK*

K. H. Figures, BDS, FDSRCS(Edin)
*Director, School of Dental Hygiene, Sheffield Health
Authority, UK*

D. J. Lamb, MDS, BDS, FDSRCS(Eng)
*Senior Lecturer and Consultant in Restorative
Dentistry, University of Sheffield, UK*

Wright

Wright
An imprint of Butterworth-Heinemann Ltd
Linacre House, Jordan Hill, Oxford OX2 8DP

 PART OF REED INTERNATIONAL BOOKS

OXFORD   LONDON   BOSTON
MUNICH   NEW DELHI   SINGAPORE   SYDNEY
TOKYO   TORONTO   WELLINGTON

First published 1992

British Library Cataloguing in Publication Data
Walsh, T. F.
  Clinical dental hygiene.
  I. Title   II. Figures, K. H.   III. Lamb, D. J.
  617.601

ISBN 0 7236 2279 5

Library of Congress Cataloguing in Publication Data
Walsh, T. F.
  Clinical dental hygiene: a handbook for the dental team/T. F.
  Walsh, K. H. Figures, D. J. Lamb.
  p. cm.
  Includes bibliographical references and index.
  ISBN 0 7236 2279 5
  1. Dental hygiene.   I. Figures, K. H.   II. Lamb, D. J. (David
  John)   III. Title.
  [DNLM: 1. Dental Care – methods – handbooks.   2. Mouth Diseases –
  handbooks.   WU 39 W227c]
  RK60.7.W37   1992
  G17.6'01–dc20
  DNLM/DLC
  for Library of Congress   91–46634
                                                                 CIP

Printed and bound in Great Britain by Redwood Press, Melksham, Wiltshire

Contents

Foreword

I am honoured to have been asked to write a foreword to this excellent book. Its authors, who are all highly respected in their field, have written a work which takes account of the profound changes which are taking place in dental education and practice. No longer does the dentist work in isolation; rather he or she is now the leader of a team, each member of which has defined but overlapping roles. Equally, dental and oral diseases are no longer perceived as separate from other diseases and all members of the dental team must be responsive to the need for whole patient care. While the necessity for all members of the profession to acquire and practise technical skills of a high order remains undiminished, there is an ever increasing additional requirement for expertise in educational methods and communication skills, with a major emphasis on prevention rather than solely on the treatment of existing disease. Finally, patterns of disease are changing throughout the world and will continue to change. It is, therefore, vital that as members of a Learned Profession we are all sensitive to new developments.

The authors have successfully dealt with the challenge of these developments and have written a book which teaches clearly and comprehensively how to maintain dental health under all conditions. I congratulate them on a splendid achievement and commend this book without reservation to all members of the dental team and others who may have any interest in oral and dental health.

H. D. Glenwright
Senior Lecturer in Periodontics
University of Birmingham

Preface

When writing this book it was our intention for it to fulfil a dual role, namely to act as a clinical text for dental hygienists and at the same time be of value to the whole dental team when confronted with problems relating to dental hygiene. It is our hope that the dental hygienist and the dental surgeon will find the content of practical worth in their day to day contacts with patients and that the dental health educator, dental surgery assistant and practice manager will also find it of use in their management of patients.

Dental hygiene is an area in which there has been considerable development in recent years and this text attempts to integrate the information in a logical and comprehensive manner.

Clinical techniques and objectives change as dental research highlights different priorities and textbooks become out of date as a result. We hope that our readers will feel that our advice is up to date and represents a consensus of current methods of use in improving the health of their patients.

TFW
KHF
DJL

Acknowledgements

The authors acknowledge their debt to Mr A. C. Crosby FRCS, Consultant in Accident and Emergency Medicine at the Royal Hallamshire Hospital, Sheffield for his advice when preparing the chapter on emergencies, and to Ron Cousins of the Clinical Illustration Department for his assistance and advice with the photography.

Part One Health

Chapter 1

Topographical and applied oral anatomy

The mouth serves to grasp, comminute and ingest food, and helps the processes of verbal and non-verbal communication by contributing to the muscles of facial expression. It is the site for the sense of taste, helps in the production and modification of speech sounds and, with the nasal cavity, provides the airway to and from the lungs. As a result it is a highly specialized organ whose complex topographical anatomy reflects the diverse activities that it must perform.

It is important that anyone advising on oral hygiene or performing clinical hygiene procedures within the mouth is aware of the anatomy of the area. To simplify the study of the topographical anatomy of the oral cavity its constituent parts will be examined in turn.

Lips and cheeks

The lips are muscular structures surrounding the commissure of the mouth. Externally they are covered with skin which is tightly bound down to the underlying connective tissue and muscle, and contains sweat glands, hair follicles and sebaceous glands. The upper lip is bounded above by the base of the nose and laterally by the nasolabial groove, a variably deep furrow passing downwards and laterally from the lateral border of the ala of the nose to a point about 1 cm lateral to the commissure of the mouth (Figure 1.1).

The lateral border of the lower lip is a less well marked furrow passing in a downwards and lateral direction from the corner of the mouth, medial to the termination of the nasolabial groove. Inferiorly, the lip is demarcated from the chin by another furrow, concave downwards, the labiomental groove. While variably deep, the nasolabial and labiomental grooves tend to become more marked with age.

The skin of the external surface of the lips and the mucous membrane of the inner surface of the lips are separated by a transitional area, the vermilion zone, which is sharply demarcated from the skin. The vermilion zone is the surface of contact between the upper and lower lip and is characterized by thin, stratified epithelium covering long, slender, densely packed connective tissue papillae. The presence of numerous blood vessels in the papillae close to the surface gives the red colour to the region, a colour enhanced by

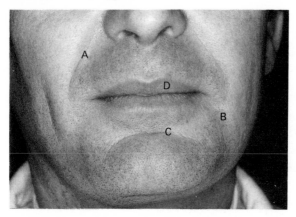

Figure 1.1 Lower third of face, showing nasolabial groove (A), groove marking lateral limit of lower lip (B), labiomental groove (C) and vermilion zone of lip (D)

the secretion of a translucent protein, eliedin, by the middle and superficial layers of epithelium. The vermilion zone contains neither hair follicles nor sweat glands, but small sebaceous glands are often present.

In the midline of the vermilion border of the upper lip there is a small tubercle, and a shallow groove – the philtrum – joins this region of the upper lip to the septum of the nose. In the average young adult the lower border of the upper lip at rest lies 1 mm or so above the incisal edges of the maxillary teeth, a relationship useful to the prosthodontist. In some cases, usually associated with mandibular retrusion, the lip line is higher and the lips incompetent. This predisposes to drying of the anterior gingivae and makes their reaction to plaque deposits more severe.

With age the depth of all furrows in the lips increases. If the teeth have been lost and overclosure occurs with decrease of the nose–chin distance, the labiomental groove deepens excessively. In some cases the folding at the corner of the mouth leads to wetting of the skin surface with saliva. Angular cheilitis can then follow with infection of the macerated skin surface by bacteria. After culture of swabs taken from the area, staphylococci from the anterior nares or *Candida albicans* from ill-cleansed dentures are commonly isolated.

The inner surface of the lips is covered with stratified squamous epithelium, tightly bound down to the underlying connective tissue and muscle. The epithelium is thin, and through it the underlying blood vessels are visible. The surface is irregular, the slight prominences being due to the presence of large numbers of small mixed salivary glands. Occasionally the ducts of such glands can become obstructed due to trauma and a mucocele results – a small saliva-filled swelling which finally ruptures either spontaneously or after being bitten.

Like the lips, the mucous membrane of the cheeks is tightly bound down to the underlying connective tissue and muscle. To allow for stretching and accommodation to the movements of mouth and cheeks, the mucous membrane has a finely wrinkled form in the resting state. Superiorly and inferiorly the boundaries of the inner surface of the cheek are the buccal sulci

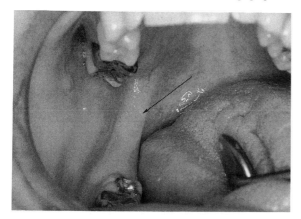

Figure 1.2   Arrow indicates pterygomandibular raphe

of the maxillary and mandibular alveolar processes. Posteriorly, the ptery-gomandibular raphe – a fibrous tissue band – stretches from the pterygoid process to the retromolar pad of the mandible (Figure 1.2). Anteriorly the mucous membrane is continuous with that of the lips.

In the maxillary second molar region the mucous membrane of the cheeks is pierced by a duct – the parotid duct – which ends as a papilla of variable size (Figure 1.3). To prevent entry of air into the duct the terminal centimetre has a valve-like form. In this final part of its course into the mouth the duct penetrates the buccinator muscle and then travels forwards for a short distance before finally penetrating the mucous membrane of the cheek.

Further down in the cheek, level with the occlusal surfaces of the teeth, there is often a slightly raised, horizontal whitish band. This is a band of keratinization produced by chronic trauma from the teeth. While sometimes barely noticeable, at other times it can be pronounced and lead to confusion with other, pathological, types of white lesion. Posteriorly and in line with the corners of the mouth there are often a small number of ectopic sebaceous glands. These are of no significance but can be alarming when present in large numbers. At times much of the cheek can be covered by such seba-

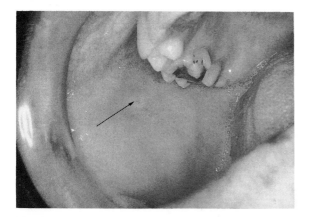

Figure 1.3   Buccal mucosa of right cheek. Arrow indicates papilla of parotid duct

ceous glands which appear as yellowish spots – Fordyce's spots – and can cause anxiety in a nervous patient when discovered for the first time.

In children the buccal fat pad can cause diagnostic problems. This is the anterior projection of a fatty covering of the muscles of mastication which projects into the cheek as a biconvex disc, of variable size, anterior to the masseter and superficial to the buccinator. While having a definite fibrous capsule its function is obscure but may provide support for the infant's cheek during suckling. A well-developed buccal fat pad can have the same appearance as an infection of the cheek.

Superiorly and inferiorly, the mucous membrane which is bound down to the underlying muscle loses its attachment and is reflected onto the bone of the alveolar processes. The zone of reflection – the sulcus – must allow for the mobility of the cheeks and the mucous membrane is attached to the underlying structures only by loose connective tissue. The sulci are horseshoe-shaped and divided into buccal and labial sections related to the cheeks and lips respectively. Where the sections join, their continuity is interrupted by a variable number of sickle-shaped fraenal attachments. The most consistently present of these are in the upper midline (Figure 1.4), which is usually well developed, and the lower midline, which is less so. Smaller fraenal attachments are usually found in the upper and lower sulci in the canine/premolar region (Figure 1.5). Fraenal attachments do not contain muscle and consist of only mucous membrane separated by a little thin fibrous tissue.

The upper midline fraenal attachment may be enlarged and have a fibrous insertion into the maxilla which, if it is associated with lack of bony fusion, may be an orthodontic problem. The remainder are of no significance in the dentate patient but may be a problem for the edentulous patient. If the denture base has to be deeply notched to provide relief over the fraenum, the notch might be judged to be a structural weakness. The fraenal attachment may then be surgically removed.

Alveolar processes

The mucous membrane covering the alveolar processes is of two types. That

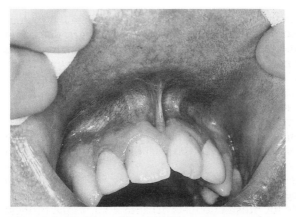

Figure 1.4   Maxillary midline labial fraenum

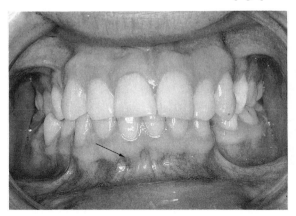

Figure 1.5 Fraenal attachments in the premolar regions. Arrow indicates the mucogingival junction between alveolar mucosa and gingivae. The alveolar prominences over the roots of the teeth are well marked

part which is continuous with the sulcus – the alveolar mucosa – is thin and loosely attached to the underlying bone by thin connective tissue. Its loose attachment permits it to accommodate to the free movement of the lips and cheeks and allows the painless deposition of local anaesthetic into the underlying connective tissue. The thinness and the plentiful blood supply give it a red colour.

In health the alveolar mucosa is separated by a scalloped line – the mucogingival junction (Figure 1.5) – from a band of thicker tissues – the gingivae – which show keratosis or parakeratosis and surround the teeth in a band approximately 5 mm thick. The more peripheral part – the attached gingivae – is bound down firmly by strong bands of collagen to the underlying alveolar bone and shows a stippling or 'orange peel' effect where the crossing over of the rete ridges causes tiny indentations of the surface. The stippling is more marked if the degree of keratosis is increased by abrasion and is noticeable in patients with good toothbrushing habits or those who have a fibrous diet.

In a Caucasian subject, healthy attached gingivae are pale pink in colour and may be demarcated by a fine depressed line from a narrow band of gingivae surrounding the teeth called the marginal or free gingivae. This surrounds the teeth, is not attached by collagen bundles to the underlying bone and hence shows little stippling. The free gingivae are also usually a rather deeper pink colour, the colour turning to the red of chronic marginal gingivitis when plaque accumulates.

The free gingivae form the interproximal papillae and, passing between the teeth as the interdental col, are continuous with the free gingivae of the other side. Behind the papilla distal to the last mandibular molar tooth lies a small glandular structure covered by loosely attached mucosa – the retromolar pad (Figure 1.6). After extraction of the mandibular teeth and the healing that follows, the residual landmark is called the pear-shaped pad. This structure is a guide for prosthodontists because it marks the furthest extension distally of a mandibular denture. It is composed of two distinct

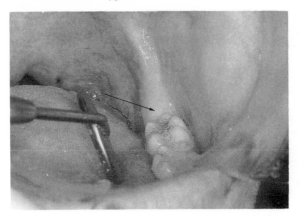

Figure 1.6   Arrow indicates retromolar pad

entities, anteriorly the remnants of the papilla and behind it the compressible retromolar pad.

The buccal and labial surfaces of the alveolar processes show a series of prominences over the roots of standing teeth (Figure 1.5). Such prominences are greatest at the cervical margins but taper towards the apices where they are undetectable. In the maxilla, those associated with the canines are usually the most marked and the central incisors less so with the prominence over the lateral incisor barely visible. In the mandible, again the canines are most prominent with the incisor prominences being smaller and of approximately equal size. The roots of the premolar and molar teeth of either jaw have a much smaller influence on topographic anatomy.

Floor of mouth and tongue

On the lingual side of the mandibular alveolar process the attached mucosa surrounding the teeth changes to loosely attached alveolar mucosa which is reflected from the bone onto the ventral surface of the tongue, so forming the lingual sulcus and the floor of the mouth. The lingual sulcus is horseshoe-shaped. Before it enters the pharynx its distal extremity is marked by a slight elevation caused by an underlying slip of the superior constrictor muscle (Figure 1.7) This small part of the muscle takes its origin on the lingual surface of the mandible just below the attachment of the pterygomandibular raphe and passes medially to its insertion in the tongue. The boundary is of interest to prosthodontists in that it marks the distal limit of the lingual flange of a mandibular denture.

From its most distal point the lingual sulcus runs forwards as a channel bounded medially by the hyoglossus muscle and laterally by the origin of the mylohyoid muscle, widens to form the floor of the mouth and ends at the midline lingual fraenum. In the floor of the mouth runs a fold which increases in size postero/anteriorly and contains the submandibular duct. The fold runs over a slight mound in the premolar region which marks the site of the sublingual gland. The ducts of the sublingual gland mostly enter the submandibular duct as it passes over its surface. The submandibular duct

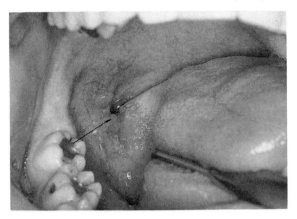

Figure 1.7 Posterior lingual sulcus with an arrow indicating the elevation marking the boundary with the pharynx and produced by the presence of a small slip of superior constrictor

and its overlying fold of mucosa passes further forwards until it ends close to the midline in a papilla, in the centre of which is the duct orifice. With the tongue raised the midline fraenum is tensed and the right and left papillae can be seen as swellings on either side of the midline (Figure 1.8). Sometimes the midline fraenum is short and tight, binding down the tip of the tongue and giving rise to a 'tongue tie'. The condition does not often give rise to functional difficulties, although at one time surgical removal was a common recommendation. Occasionally it makes cleaning the lingual surfaces of the mandibular anterior teeth difficult, when its removal may be more rationally indicated.

The undersurface of the tongue is marked by several fimbriae or folds and is covered by squamous epithelium. Beneath the thin mucosa, tortuous, bluish veins are often visible. The marked tortuosity allows for accommodation to the movements of the tongue.

The dorsal surface of the tongue is divided into two zones. The anterior two-thirds is separated from the posterior third by a V-shaped groove – the

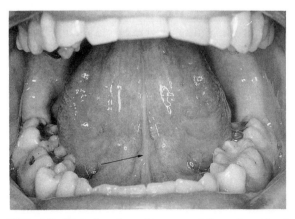

Figure 1.8 Ventral surface of tongue and floor of mouth. Arrow indicates papilla of right submandibular duct

terminal sulcus – the apex pointing backwards. Several types of papillae are visible. Immediately anterior to the terminal sulcus is a line of large, mushroom-shaped circumvallate papillae, the larger nearer the midline. Each is surrounded by a trough containing taste buds. Much of the remainder of the anterior dorsal surface is covered with filiform and fungiform papillae. The filiform are the more numerous, each being hair-like, keratinized and surrounding the shorter, mushroom-like fungiform papillae. The fungiform papillae have a thinner coating of epithelium and are correspondingly more red in colour. They contain variable numbers of taste buds. On the lateral border of the tongue, posteriorly, can be found a few foliate papillae containing numerous taste buds. In man the foliate papillae are insignificant but they are present in considerable numbers in those animals with a well developed sense of taste.

A marked central fissure is often characteristic of the anterior two-thirds of the dorsum of tongue, and at the apex of the V-shaped groove separating the anterior and posterior parts of the tongue a small blind pit – the foramen caecum – marks the point from which the developing thyroid gland descends into the neck.

The posterior third of the tongue is pale pink and faces back into the pharynx. It is covered with lingual follicles, which are low prominences containing lymphoid tissue and surrounded by shallow furrows. The sum total of the lymphoid tissue in the posterior third of the tongue is called the lingual tonsil.

Hard palate, soft palate and pharynx

The hard palate forms the roof of the mouth and, having an accessory part to play in mastication, is covered with keratinized epithelium. Peripherally it is covered with mucoperiosteum continuous with the attached gingivae, and attached firmly to the underlying bone. More centrally, in the angle between the palatine and alveolar processes of the maxilla, it is separated from the bone by intervening connective tissue containing blood vessels and nerves. The presence of connective tissue between the epithelium and bone allows anaesthetic to be infiltrated without causing pain. Further centrally and in the midline the epithelium is again tightly bound down to the underlying bone, which is sometimes raised in the midline as a midline palatal torus of variable size.

In the midline, posterior to the central incisor teeth, lies the incisive papilla, an oval prominence covering the incisal fossa and marking the entry into the mouth of the nasopalatine nerves. The incisive papilla serves as a useful landmark when attempting to anaesthetize the nerve supply to the soft tissues lingual to the maxillary central incisor teeth. Just distal to the incisive papilla are a variable number of roughly parallel irregular raised folds of mucoperiosteum – the palatal rugae – which in lower animals have a more important accessory role to play in mastication (Figure 1.9). Even further posteriorly, marking the junction of hard and soft palate, lie two small indentations, one on either side of the midline. These are the foveae palatini, where the ducts of two small clusters of salivary glands open into the mouth.

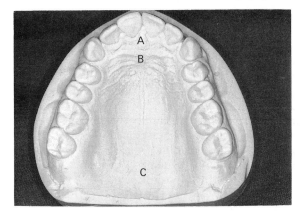

Figure 1.9 Model cast from impression of palatal surface of maxilla: A, incisive papilla; B, rugae; C, approximate position of foveae palatini

The soft palate is covered with stratified squamous epithelium and divides the oropharynx from the nasopharynx. It terminates distally in a short muscular projection – the uvula – and by its contact with the posterior wall of the pharynx regulates the flow of air through the mouth and nose when breathing and speaking. At this point on the posterior wall of the pharynx a functional thickening of the superior constrictor muscle, called the ridge of Passavant, aids production of an air-tight seal.

Laterally the side of the pharynx is marked by two arches. The anterior is produced by the presence of the palatoglossus muscle. It is separated by the pharyngeal tonsil from the distal arch, which is formed by the palatopharyngeus muscle (Figure 1.10). The pharyngeal tonsil is a collection of lymph tissue and in young patients is frequently red and swollen in response to infection. In later life it atrophies and even shows calcification, which can be a source of diagnostic confusion on panoramic radiographs. The pharyngeal tonsil is part of a ring of lymphoid tissue, the other parts of which are the

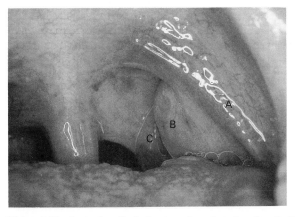

Figure 1.10 Lateral wall of pharynx: A, palatoglossal arch; B, pharyngeal tonsil; C, palatopharyngeal arch

lingual tonsil, found on the posterior third of the tongue, and the adenoids, a collection of lymph tissue found in the midline of the posterior wall of the nasopharynx.

Chapter 2

Topographical and applied dental anatomy

The clinical crown

A tooth may be divided into crown and root, the crown being covered by enamel and the root by cementum. The two surfaces meet at the cement–enamel junction which is visible as the cervical line on the neck of the tooth. In the healthy mouth of a young adult the level of gingival attachment will be coronal to the cervical line. The anatomical crown ends at the cervical line, in contrast to the clinical crown which is the amount of tooth protruding beyond the gingival margin into the patient's mouth (Figure 2.1). Variations

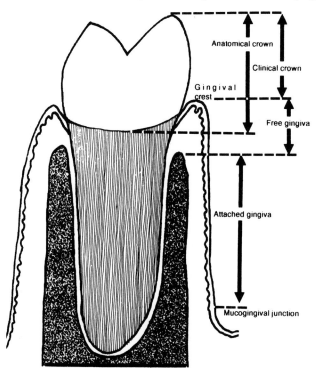

Figure 2.1 The anatomical surface landmarks of the tooth and gingival tissues

in clinical crown length are often produced by different levels of gingival attachment to the tooth and are seen in patients suffering from gingival recession and hence showing increased clinical crown length. Short clinical crowns are seen in teeth that have worn excessively, commonly due to bruxism, or where only a few teeth remain which, as a consequence, have been worn down due to concentrated attrition.

Although many oral hygiene procedures influence the condition and health of the oral soft tissues, it is towards the dental hard tissues that they are primarily directed. This chapter will concentrate on those aspects of the dental hard tissues which are of relevance to the dental worker concerned with clinical dental hygiene.

Incisors and canines have four axial surfaces converging in an incisal edge. Premolars and molars have five surfaces the incisal edge being replaced by an occlusal surface. The surface of the crown shows many elevations and depressions which make up the typical appearance of the tooth. The following terms are used in the description of crown anatomy:

Cusp: an elevation or mound on the occlusal surface.
Cingulum: the lingual convex bulge on an anterior tooth.
Tubercle: a small elevation on some part of the crown produced by an extra formation of enamel and dentine. These are quite frequently seen buccally on deciduous first molars (the tubercle of Zuckerkandl) and lingually on upper first molars (the cusp of Carabelli).
Ridge: a linear elevation on the surface of a tooth. A good example is the marginal ridge found on the mesial and distal surfaces of molars and premolars.
Fissure: an irregular linear depression in the tooth surface. A pit is a small pinpoint depression.
Developmental groove: a developmental deformity in the crown and/or root of a tooth. This type of defect will encourage the formation of a periodontal pocket, particularly when it involves the root, because dental plaque will collect there undisturbed. Grooves are sometimes seen on permanent upper lateral incisors, especially on palatal surfaces.
Mamelon: any one of the three rounded protuberances found on the incisal edges of recently erupted anterior teeth. Mamelons wear away quickly, usually within 2 years of eruption.
Facet: a small, smooth, flat surface seen on the occlusal aspect of the crown indicating an abnormal pattern of wear on the enamel.
Perikymata: seen commonly on recently erupted incisors as a series of horizontal ridges running parallel to the incisal edge and quite often affecting the whole of the labial surface of the crown.

Primary dentition

The eruption of the primary teeth begins at about 6 months of age with the mandibular incisors. All primary teeth have usually erupted by the age of 2 years, although there is considerable individual variation with some children not exhibiting their first tooth until they are over 1 year old. There do not appear to be any ethnic differences in the dates of eruption but severe

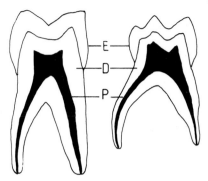

Figure 2.2 Comparison of primary and permanent molar teeth. The primary molar has thinner enamel (E) and dentine (D), but larger pulp chamber (P)

malnutrition may cause delayed eruption as well as seriously affecting other aspects of the child's growth.

The usual order of appearance of the primary teeth in the mouth is:

1. Central incisors.
2. Lateral incisors.
3. First molars.
4. Canines.
5. Second molars.

Mandibular teeth usually erupt before maxillary teeth. As the child approaches the age of 5 years, spacing will appear between the deciduous teeth as a result of the jaw growth required to accommodate the developing permanent teeth (Figure 2.2).

Permanent dentition

Eruption of the mandibular permanent teeth tends to occur slightly ahead of the maxillary, by a few months. Some studies have shown boys to have

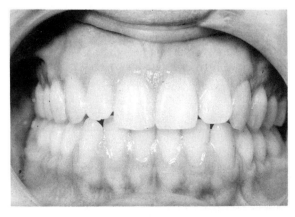

Figure 2.3 An ideal dentition in a 20 year old: perfect occlusion, no restorations and healthy gingival condition

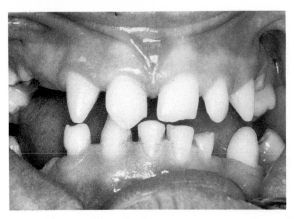

Figure 2.4 Dental hypodontia: many permanent teeth are missing and those present are of poor quality and shape

delayed eruption compared with girls. Interestingly, black children in the USA show slightly earlier eruption dates compared with Caucasians. This has also been shown to be true when African blacks are compared with European Caucasian subjects. Only the permanent molars erupt without displacing a primary predecessor and the first permanent molar appears at the age of 6 years (Figure 2.3).

The loss of the primary teeth is due to resorption of their roots associated with the progressive eruption of their permanent successors. The resorption is undertaken by odontoclasts and proceeds intermittently so that a certain amount of repair occurs simultaneously. Sometimes, shedding is delayed, resulting in a permanent incisor erupting lingually to the primary one. More rarely, fusion of the primary tooth to alveolar bone may develop. This ankylosis of tooth to bone is most often seen in primary second molars which have no permanent successor or in teeth such as maxillary primary canines when they are ectopically placed.

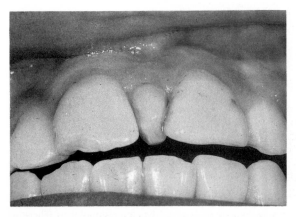

Figure 2.5 A mesiodens: a supernumerary tooth lying between the upper central incisors

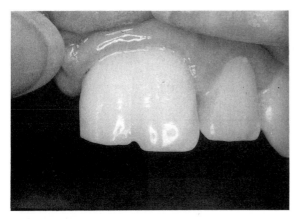

Figure 2.6 Fused upper central incisors

Developmental variations in the dentition

Hypodontia

This mainly affects the permanent teeth and it is not unusual to find one or more teeth missing (Figure 2.4). The teeth most commonly absent are, in order of frequency: third molars, maxillary lateral incisors and second premolars. This condition may also be a result of a local disorder such as cleft palate or of many systemic disorders. Ectodermal dysplasia is a condition where many primary and secondary teeth are missing together with other abnormalities such as lack of eyebrows, sparse hair growth and a lack of sweat glands.

Hyperdontia
Additional or supernumary teeth usually have a rudimentary shape, often conical, and are most commonly seen in the maxillary incisor region where,

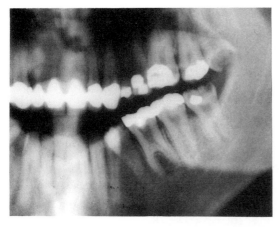

Figure 2.7 Radiograph of a patient with taurodontism. The elongated roots of 36 and 37 demonstrate this

if one is present in the midline, it is called a mesiodens (Figure 2.5). They can affect the eruption of neighbouring teeth and may be the source of cyst formation. When erupted they may cause plaque stagnation. A supplemental tooth is an extra tooth which exactly mirrors one already present. Supernumary teeth are also seen in systemic disorders such as cleidocranial dysostosis.

Gemination
This is the result of the incomplete division of a tooth germ and is most commonly seen in the incisor region when a central and lateral incisor may be joined to form one large tooth with a common root. A groove marking the junction is quite often seen in the crown of such a tooth.

Fusion
This occurs when two tooth germs fuse to form one large tooth (Figure 2.6). It is often difficult to tell the difference between fusion and gemination and so the term 'twinned tooth' is often used.

Odontome
An odontome is any developmental malformation of dental tissues and a tooth exhibiting gemination may also be called a geminated odontome. An invaginated odontome is seen quite often on maxillary lateral incisors where a deep pit forms on the palatal surface due to a defect in the tooth germ. On a radiograph the tooth resembles a tooth within a tooth. This deep pit is very susceptible to caries.

Taurodontism
Teeth that exhibit this condition lack a pronounced cervical line and have parallel sided roots (Figure 2.7). The pulp chambers are enlarged in an apical direction and second permanent molars are commonly affected.

Enamel nodule or pearl
This is a small circular lump of enamel (and dentine) found near the cervical line which may be mistaken for subgingival calculus (Figure 2.8).

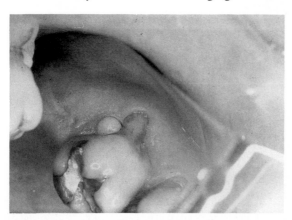

Figure 2.8 An enamel pearl visible at the gingival margin of an upper molar

Part Two   Disease

Chapter 3

Oral pathology

Oral mucosa

Ulcers and bullous conditions

The most common disorder to affect the oral mucosa is ulceration, but the cause is often obscure. An ulcer may be defined as a break in the continuity of surface epithelium. Before examining an ulcer the clinician will check whether the patient is aware of any previous trauma to the area and how long it has been present. Its size and position are noted together with the type of margin it presents. An ulcer with a raised, rolled and everted margin is often malignant and palpation of the regional lymph nodes may be undertaken before the ulcer is examined in detail. Ulceration may influence oral hygiene in two ways: its presence may hinder cleaning but also careful control of the adjacent oral flora will, by reducing secondary infection, help to speed healing. Some of the more common types of oral ulceration will now be described.

Traumatic ulcer
A traumatic ulcer can be produced as a result of physical, chemical or thermal injury. Examples of physical trauma include biting the mucosa, denture irritation, toothbrush injury or a sharp edge of a broken tooth. The once common practice of placing an aspirin tablet next to a painful tooth will give rise to a chemical burn as may careless use of acid etchant solutions (Figure 3.1). Thermal injury may be caused by any hot substances entering the mouth. Traumatic ulcers will heal rapidly once the source of trauma is removed, followed by the use for a few days of chlorhexidine mouthwash, which will help to reduce the level of secondary infection of the ulcerated surface. Benzydamine mouthwash is also often helpful in relieving the discomfort produced by a traumatic ulcer. Rarely, ulceration is self-inflicted. Such patients obviously have a psychiatric problem and are reluctant to admit causing the lesion.

Recurrent aphthous ulceration (RAU)
This is a common form of oral ulceration characterized by the development of painful and recurrent lesions which most commonly occur between the ages of 10 and 30 years and more frequently in females. It has been said that

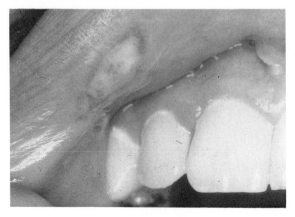

Figure 3.1　A chemical burn on the mucosa of the upper lip caused by acid etchant solution

nearly 20% of the population have experienced these at some stage of their lives. They can vary in size from 2 mm to over 1 cm in diameter and are most common on non-keratinized mucosa such as buccal, labial and floor of mouth mucosa. The ulcers may persist for over 10 days before gradually healing. Recurrent aphthae are classified into three groups based upon their clinical manifestations; these are: minor aphthae, major aphthae and herpetiform aphthae.

Minor aphthae account for 80% of cases (Figure 3.2), with major aphthae accounting for only 10% (Figure 3.3). The difference between minor and major is that major aphthae can take several weeks to heal and tend to affect the posterior part of the mouth and keratinized mucosa. In recent years major aphthae have been added to the list of changes which may indicate HIV infection. Herpetiform aphthae, which also account for 10% of RAU, are more commonly seen in females and present as multiple small ulcers (Figure 3.4) which coalesce to form large areas of irregular ulceration. They have a similar healing time to minor aphthae.

So far no single causative factor of RAU has been found although a number of associated conditions are often present. There is little doubt that

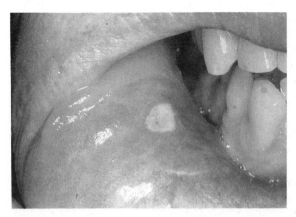

Figure 3.2　A minor aphthous ulcer which had been present for 5 days

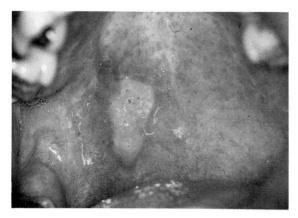

Figure 3.3 A major aphthous ulcer on the soft palate which had been present for 3 weeks

RAU is associated with deficiency states and a full haematological measurement of haemoglobin, ferritin, vitamin B_{12} and corrected whole blood folate should be routine. Deficiency states are not diseases in themselves but are a result of either reduced dietary intake, poor gut absorption or excessive blood loss. Anaemia can cause oral ulceration and sideropenia (iron deficiency anaemia) in women is usually associated with menorrhagia, whereas deficiencies of folic acid or vitamin B_{12} are suggestive of the presence of coeliac disease or pernicious anaemia, respectively.

It would appear that anxiety or stress are important factors in people who suffer from RAU. Ulcers commonly appear at examination times in school and college students. Furthermore, some foodstuffs, in particular chocolate and preservatives, may induce RAU and if this is thought to be the case then patch testing to detect potential allergens would be appropriate.

Treatment of RAU depends on obtaining a good history to specifically exclude allergies, and then to undertake haematological investigations. While waiting for the results of these investigations, the use of chlorhexidine mouthwash or gel applied to the ulcer is beneficial or, alternatively, benzydamine mouthwash can be used. Limiting the intake of crisps and carbo-

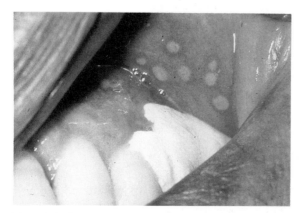

Figure 3.4 Herpetiform aphthae, adjacent to a periodontal dressing

nated drinks is to be recommended. Careful plaque control procedures also need to be started to avoid trauma during toothbrushing and the patient should be counselled to maintain good oral hygiene, especially in the vicinity of ulcers, in order to reduce secondary contamination by dental plaque. Some patients benefit from the use of topical steroid therapy in the form of hydrocortisone (2.5 mg pellet) allowed to dissolve next to the ulcer three times daily. Some clinicians also prescribe Adcortyl in Orabase, a topical preparation of triamcinolone in emollient, which can be applied to the ulcer directly. Information on any abnormalities of the blood picture should be passed on to the patient's physician for appropriate treatment.

Ulcers produced by viruses
Two groups of viruses are responsible for the majority of viral conditions that present to the dental clinician, namely herpes and Coxsackie viruses. Herpes simplex virus type 1 is responsible for primary herpetic gingivostomatitis (Figure 3.5). More recently a second herpes virus, known as type II, has been identified which was originally associated with genital infections but is now increasingly involved in oral infections. Herpes type 1 infection is endemic and, by the age of 12 years, 40% of children have antibody to the virus; this rises to 90% in adults reaching the age of 60 years. Initial infection may be mild producing very few symptoms or it may be quite severe, with general widespread oral ulceration producing extreme difficulty in eating or talking and also in cleaning teeth. There is a marked cervical lymphadenopathy in these severe cases together with a general feeling of being unwell. The herpes lesion starts initially as a minute vesicle but this soon ruptures to produce an ulcer which can be present on keratinized or non-keratinized mucosa. Treatment depends on the severity at the time of presentation. Severe cases may need specific antiviral therapy in the form of acyclovir either as an elixir for children or tablets for adults (200 mg five times daily). Patients should be advised to use an antiseptic mouthwash such as 0.2% chlorhexidine gluconate to reduce plaque levels. Previous experience shows that, in the absence of treatment, the ulcers will have healed within 10–14 days.

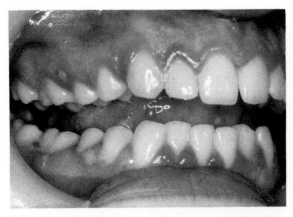

Figure 3.5   Primary herpetiform gingivostomatitis with characteristic ulcers present throughout the mouth together with acute gingivitis

The other viral conditions which may produce oral ulceration are less common and less severe. Herpangina, which is seen in children, is caused by viruses of the coxsackie group and commonly affects the posterior part of the mouth. The condition is only mild and treatment is to use an antiseptic mouthwash. Hand, foot and mouth disease is also usually seen in childhood although adults may be affected. It is caused by Coxsackie type A16 virus and the clinical manifestations are of multiple shallow oral ulcers together with erythematous macules on the hands and feet. Treatment is symptomatic with the use of chlorhexidine mouthwash to reduce plaque contamination of the oral ulcers.

Bullous conditions affecting the oral mucosa
The conditions which may produce a bulla on the oral mucosa also often affect the skin. A bulla is a large fluid-filled vesicle or blister and can be intraepithelial or subepithelial. Pemphigus vulgaris is a chronic bulla-forming disease of skin and oral mucosa with a deteriorating prognosis and an autoimmune cause. In 60% of patients the presenting symptoms occur in the mouth (Figure 3.6). In this condition the bullae develop within the epithelium and tend to rupture shortly after formation leaving a non-specific ulceration which sometimes makes it difficult to arrive at a correct diagnosis. However, immunofluorescence microscopy will reveal antibody deposition within the epithelium. Benign mucous membrane pemphigoid is another bullous disease but here the bullae form in the connective tissue immediately beneath the epithelium. It is rare to find this disease in men but women over the age of 50 appear to be more prone to it. By means of immunofluorescence microscopy it can be demonstrated that the basement membrane is the site of immunoglobulins which appear to be attacking this structure.

White patches

The majority of white patches seen in the mouth are benign, but certain conditions may be premalignant or malignant. Unfortunately, it is often

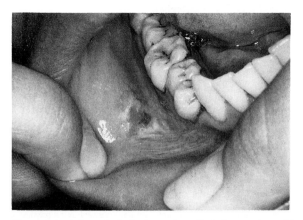

Figure 3.6   A burst bulla in the oral vestibule in a patient with pemphigus vulgaris

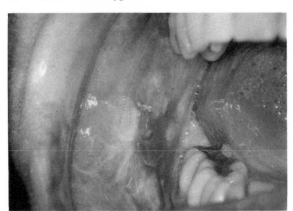

Figure 3.7   An aspirin burn which has produced ulceration and a white patch in the buccal mucosa adjacent to the last molar

difficult to decide clinically which are the sinister lesions and therefore a biopsy of all white patches is required. However, when a white patch is discovered in the mouth the first step is to identify any possible traumatic cause such as cheek biting or placing an aspirin tablet next to a painful tooth (Figure 3.7). Chronic denture irritation will give rise to a thickening of the mucosa at the site of trauma and also patients who do not wear dentures may show hyperkeratosis of the mucosa covering the ridges due to the effect of mastication without teeth. Nicotinic stomatitis or smoker's keratosis may give rise to white patch formation particularly in the palate. This is more commonly seen in pipe smokers and although the condition is not considered to be premalignant its presence should be an indication to stop smoking (Figure 3.8). It is rare for a squamous cell carcinoma to develop on the palate but if a lesion is present for more than 2 weeks then further investigation should be undertaken.

Besides trauma, candidal infection may produce white patches and the

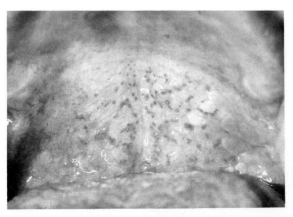

Figure 3.8   Stomatitis nicotina on the palate of a pipe smoker. The hard palate has a hyperkeratotic appearance with red spots which are the openings of the minor mucous glands

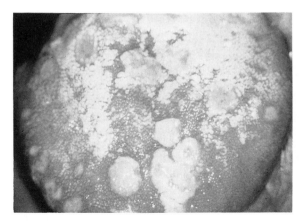

Figure 3.9   Candidal infection affecting the tongue in a patient using a steroid inhaler for asthma

two candidoses of importance in this respect are acute pseudomembranous candidosis (thrush) and chronic hyperplastic candidosis. Patients taking broad-spectrum antibiotics or receiving steroid therapy, particularly via inhalers, may have acute pseudomembranous candidosis (Figure 3.9), but in others an immunological deficiency such as neutropenia or undiagnosed diabetes mellitus may be the cause. HIV infection may be another reason for the presence of thrush. Chronic hyperplastic candidosis characteristically occurs in the commissure region and is frequently seen bilaterally as a well defined area of redness of the mucosa with associated white patches (Figure 3.10). This appearance is sometimes called speckled leucoplakia. This chronic candidal condition is known to be premalignant if an effective treatment regime is not adhered to.

Recently, a new antifungal drug, fluconazole, has been found to be effective in treating chronic hyperplastic candidosis but any patient treated in this way should be maintained on long-term follow-up.

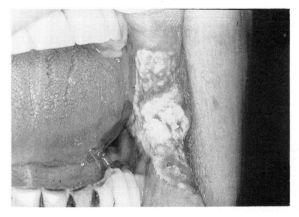

Figure 3.10   Chronic hyperplastic candidosis affecting the left commissure of the lip

Premalignant and malignant lesions of oral mucosa

The survival rate from oral cancer is only 50% after 5 years and current trends reveal an increase in the incidence of oral malignancy. Very often the first sign of neoplastic change of the oral mucosa is the appearance of a white patch. This is sometimes referred to as 'leucoplakia'. Indeed, leucoplakia can be defined as a white patch or plaque that cannot be characterized clinically or histologically as any other disease. Widespread use of this term has resulted in an association with oral malignant change and as a consequence the very use of the word leucoplakia often causes the clinician to think that sinister changes are taking place in that area of mucosa. The most significant aetiological factors in leucoplakia associated with the subsequent development of oral cancer are tobacco usage, alcohol consumption, nutritional deficiency and candidal infection. The early histological signs of oral cancer developing in the epithelium are referred to as epithelial dysplasia. This may be classified by the pathologist as mild, moderate or severe. Once the basal layer of cells has been disturbed by neoplastic change then the diagnosis of early squamous cell carcinoma (SCC) can be made.

Squamous cell carcinoma

Malignant disease may present as an oral ulcer, and squamous cell carcinoma is the commonest of all oral neoplasms forming 1% of all neoplasms (Figure 3.11). It tends to be more prevalent in the lower socioeconomic groups and its incidence is directly related to the use of tobacco and the consumption of alcohol. The chewing of betel nut or ghat has been shown to have a positive correlation. The dental clinician must be vigilant in examining the oral mucosa of each patient and the need for an early biopsy of any suspicious ulcer cannot be over-emphasized. This is one of the main reasons for maintaining the 6-monthly checkup.

Various methods of treatment of SCC are available and include surgery,

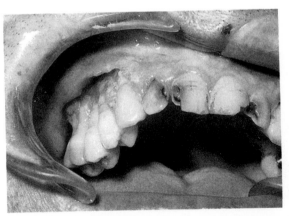

Figure 3.11 Primary squamous cell carcinoma involving the gingiva of 16, 15, 14

radiotherapy, chemotherapy, cryosurgery and laser therapy. Chemotherapy may be administered systemically or, in some cases, topically.

Lichen planus

Oral lichen planus is characterized by the presence of white patches which principally affect the buccal mucosa but the tongue, lips and attached gingiva can be affected. Lichen planus can be divided into four subtypes, reticular, erosive, plaque-like and atrophic. However, in the same patient different types may be seen at the same time in different sites. The commonest type to affect oral mucosa is the reticular variety and it can be recognized as an interlacing network of white striae which run across the buccal mucosa (Figure 3.12) and more rarely floor of mouth mucosa. The aetiology of lichen planus is unknown and at present the treatment involves the use of topical steroids in a mouth bath if symptoms are present. Lichenoid reactions do occur as a result of drug therapy, and in these patients changing the causative drug may allow the mucosa to return to normal.

Conditions affecting the tongue

Conditions affecting the tongue can be systemic or local in origin. Local conditions are commonest and these will be covered first. A common condition that may only produce a mild burning sensation of the tongue mucosa is of erythema migrans (geographical tongue), which is seen as a clearly defined area of depapillation in the dorsum of the tongue (Figure 3.13). After a week or so, this area will have returned to normal and the 'bald patch' may have moved on to involve another area of the tongue. This condition is not sinister in any way and does not require any treatment.

Another condition which is similar in appearance to erythema migrans, but the area of depapillation stays in one place, is median rhomboid glossitis

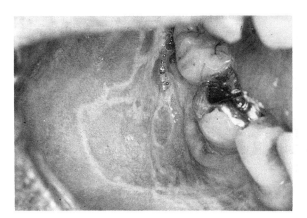

Figure 3.12   Typical reticular, 'lace' pattern seen in lichen planus

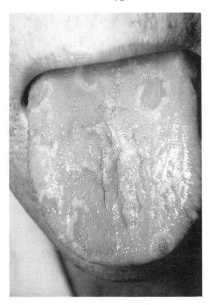

Figure 3.13   Erythema migrans or geographical tongue

(Figure 3.14). Here the 'bald patch' is located on the dorsum symmetrically placed across the centre line towards the back of the tongue. It is not clinically significant but may be associated with candidal infection which should be treated.

White patches may be seen on the tongue mucosa and those which affect the dorsum include lichen planus, which is most commonly seen as a white plaque. Squamous cell carcinoma may present initially on the tongue mucosa as a white patch and 'hairy leucoplakia' which is seen on the lateral margins of tongue is seen as one of the later changes of HIV infection (Figure 3.15). Any ulcer or white patch on the tongue should be biopsied if the cause is not obvious. It is also worth noting that the ventral surface of the

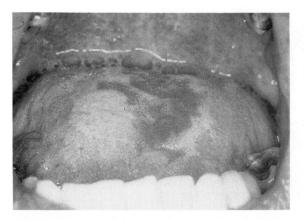

Figure 3.14   Median rhomboid glossitis

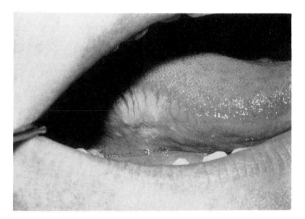

Figure 3.15 'Hairy leucoplakia' involving the lateral border of the tongue in a HIV positive patient

tongue is an area that should be carefully examined for white patches as malignant change in lesions on the floor of mouth mucosa is not unusual.

The dorsum of the tongue can also be affected in iron deficiency anaemia, resulting in a smooth surface due to the loss of papillae (Figure 3.16). This condition is more commonly seen in elderly patients who may be malnourished, or have a condition which causes blood loss such as a peptic ulcer or a malignancy. Pernicious anaemia caused by a lack of vitamin B_{12} absorption will produce a 'red beefy tongue'. Correction of the underlying anaemia by the patient's physician will allow the tongue to return to normal.

Conditions affecting the lips

The commonest conditions to affect the lips are herpes labialis (cold sore) and angular cheilitis. Herpes simplex virus type 1 is commonly responsible for the appearance of a cold sore (Figure 3.17). In this condition reactivation of the virus occurs which has remained dormant in the tissues, possibly as a

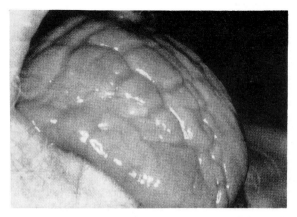

Figure 3.16 'Red beefy' tongue seen in an iron-deficient patient. There are no papillae visible on the dorsum of the tongue

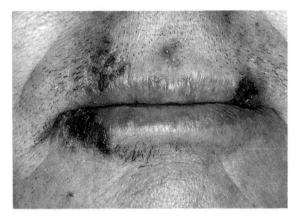

Figure 3.17   Herpes labialis or cold sores of the lip

result of trauma, exposure to sunlight, menstruation or systemic upset. The first sign of viral activity is the feeling of a 'prickling sensation' which is followed within 24 hours by the appearance of small vesicles on the lip. Acyclovir cream if applied early is effective in treating herpes labialis.

Angular cheilitis is a common condition affecting the lips and as a general rule is seen in patients who wear a dental prosthesis. This is covered in detail in Chapter 11. This condition may be seen in younger people who are dentate and a pure staphylococcal infection is often to blame. Here a depression in the host response may have occurred as this is seen more commonly in winter time but the possibility of HIV infection should be considered.

The lower lip is a common site for squamous cell carcinoma and this may appear as a small scab which fails to heal. A person who smokes or works outdoors and as a consequence is frequently exposed to sunlight is at risk of developing this condition.

Conditions affecting the gingiva

The commonest condition to affect the gingiva is inflammatory periodontal disease which is covered in Chapter 8. Many conditions can affect the gingiva and these can be classified as systemic and local. A more detailed classification of the systemic ones is shown in Table 3.1.

The systemic conditions which frequently produce changes in the gingival tissues do so by depressing the host response to plaque resulting in an exaggerated tissue inflammatory response. Acute monocytic leukaemia which is one of the rarer leukaemias is known to affect the gingival tissues and tends to be more common in young adults (Figure 3.18). The clinical appearance of the gingiva is that of marked swelling accompanied by deep pseudo-pockets, and the marginal tissue may bleed spontaneously – the bleeding being difficult to stop. Acute myeloid leukaemia can present with gingival bleeding alone and no other symptoms although there may be a mild marginal gingivitis. Except in the young patient the prognosis in acute leukaemia is poor.

Table 3.1.   Examples of the effects on the gingiva of a systemic condition or its treatment

Body system	Condition
Blood	Leukaemia, neutropenia, anaemia
Endocrine	Diabetes mellitus
Skin	Lichen planus, pemphigus, mucous membrane pemphigoid
Genitourinary	Pregnancy
Drug therapy	Phenytoin, nifedipine, cyclosporin hyperplasia

Another haematological condition which produces gingival changes is cyclic neutropenia where the number of circulating polymorphonuclear neutrophils falls dramatically every few weeks. After about 8 days the levels rise again but when the count is low the patient suffers from general malaise and pyrexia. The oral changes which occur consist of a mild gingivitis and/or aphthae-like ulcerations confined to the marginal gingivae where recurrent aphthae are rarely seen. Localized zones of hyperaemia affecting the marginal gingiva of just one tooth may also be seen.

Diabetes mellitus is a systemic condition where there has been shown to be a defect in neutrophil function. In patients with this disease varying degrees of periodontal involvement may be seen. The neutrophil disorder that has been identified is one of impaired chemotaxis and subsequent phagocytosis.

Along with the usual plaque control methods in many cases the local treatment of these conditions can be assisted by use of an antiplaque mouthwash, but treatment of the underlying systemic condition is crucial.

The local conditions which produce gingival problems include gingival epulides, overhangs from a restoration, and finally the diseases of acute necrotizing gingivitis and acute herpetic gingivostomatitis which are both covered in Chapter 9. A granulomatous epulis or a pyogenic granuloma is

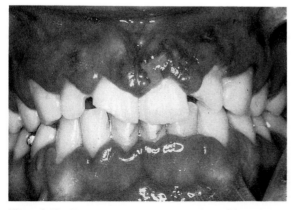

Figure 3.18   Gingival appearance of a patient with acute monocytic leukaemia. The gingival tissue is grossly swollen with ulceration and spontaneous bleeding due to low platelet levels

seen in the presence of localized chronic inflammation such as subgingival calculus or an overhang on a restoration (Figure 3.19a and b). This type of epulis is an exuberant response of the gingival tissue to the irritation and is quite commonly seen in pregnant women whose oral hygiene is poor (Figure 3.20). The treatment involves encouraging good oral hygiene and the removal of the calculus or overhangs. As soon as inflammation has subsided an excision biopsy should be performed.

There are other types of epulides but these are less common. Examples include giant cell epulis, congenital epulis and fibrous epulis. Swellings which appear on the gingivae may arise from other structures within the mouth or be related to them. Local pathology which could present as a gingival swelling includes chronic periapical pathology, odontogenic cysts and neoplasms and overt malignant disease such as squamous cell carcinoma. The possibility of a metastatic tumour in a patient who has been treated for a malignant condition should not be overlooked.

Desquamative gingivitis is the term used to describe a condition which produces a thinning of the gingival epithelium (Figure 3.21) and can be seen when lichen planus or bullous conditions affect the gingiva. In lichen planus

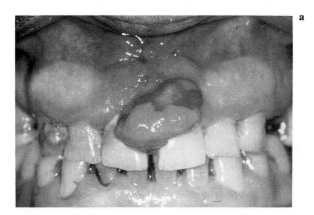

a

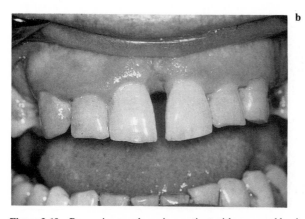

b

Figure 3.19   Pyogenic granuloma in a patient with poor oral hygiene: (a) prior to excision; (b) after excision

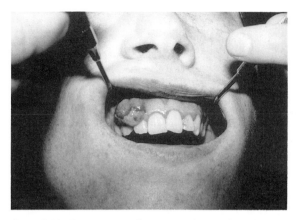

Figure 3.20 Pregnancy epulis or pyogenic granuloma in a pregnant patient. The exacerbation of the pre-existing gingivitis is also noticeable

the clinical picture is one of the gingivae appearing very red, particularly the buccal gingivae, with the lingual gingival tissue being rarely affected. This condition can be very difficult to treat as current knowledge regarding treatment is limited. Good plaque control is important and in many cases the use of a steroid-containing mouthwash and an antiseptic mouthrinse can be beneficial.

Drug-induced gingival conditions

The drugs which may produce an effect on the gingival tissues are quite varied. The most well known are the phenytoin derivatives such as Dilantin or Epanutin which are used to control epilepsy. Patients who take this drug often have gingival overgrowth (Figure 3.22) and a number of studies have tried to discover the cause of the gingival swelling. By means of autoradiog-

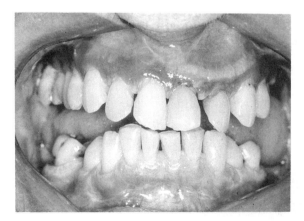

Figure 3.21 Erosive lichen planus affecting the gingival margin producing 'desquamative gingivitis'

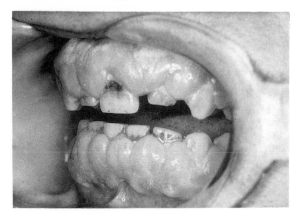

Figure 3.22   Gingival hyperplasia in an epileptic patient taking sodium phenytoin

raphy it has been shown that fibroblasts from phenytoin-conditioned gingival tissue show an increase in mitotic activity. However, the number of fibroblasts per unit of tissue is normal so it is not hyperplasia but uncontrolled fibroblast growth. Hence the condition should be more correctly termed phenytoin-induced gingival overgrowth.

Nifedipine, which is a calcium channel blocking agent, has recently been shown to produce gingival overgrowth which resembles that seen in phenytoin controlled individuals (Figure 3.23). Drugs from the same pharmacological group as nifedipine have also been shown to produce this effect. The third drug which has been found to produce gingival overgrowth is the immunosuppressant cyclosporin which is frequently taken by patients who have had a renal transplant (Figure 3.24).

The last category of drugs which may produce gingival changes are the oral contraceptives. Several studies have shown that women taking these have a higher incidence of gingivitis and an increased flow of gingival fluid.

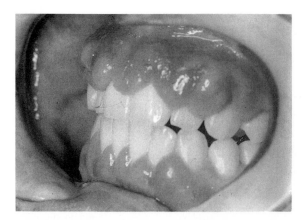

Figure 3.23   Gingival hyperplasia in a patient taking nifedipine

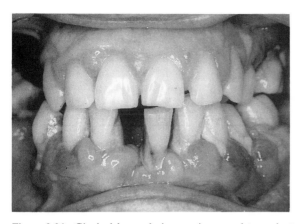

Figure 3.24   Gingival hyperplasia seen in a renal transplant patient taking cyclosporin to prevent organ rejection

Allergic reactions

Intraoral allergic reactions do occur from time to time, and these may be due to components of the diet or dentifrice constituents. Very rarely the poly-methylmethacrylate of dental appliances is incriminated (Figure 3.25). Even chemicals in impression materials or the use of rubber dam may induce a hypersensitivity reaction. The presenting signs of an oral hypersensitivity reaction are facial or lip swelling, gingivitis, oral ulceration and swelling of the oral mucosa which may have a cobblestone appearance. Not all of these signs would be present simultaneously. Also, some patients with burning mouth syndrome can be shown to have an allergic response underlying the symptoms. The dietary factors which may induce an oral response include cinnamonaldehyde and the benzoates which are designated by the E numbers E210–E219 as additives to foodstuffs. Skin patch testing by a dermatologist will identify possible allergens.

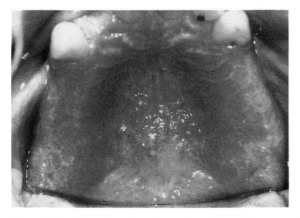

Figure 3.25   Allergy to polymethylmethacrylate which was confirmed by patch testing

Chapter 4

Dental pathology

The most significant influence on dental hygiene will be the efforts that the patient makes at removing dental plaque deposits. However, pathology of the teeth and subsequent repair of this damage will be a major factor in helping or hindering the efforts of the patient. For this reason the commoner conditions seen affecting the teeth will be described in this chapter.

Dental caries

Since the early part of this century a tremendous amount of data has been collected on the development and progression of dental caries. Most relates to the carious attack of enamel. G.V. Black stressed the importance of understanding the caries disease process and advocated definite procedures to ensure its complete eradication. His beliefs and principles of cavity preparation were followed until the 1970s when dentists began to suggest that new recommendations should be laid down. This reflected a better understanding of the disease process itself, together with the availability of effective preventive measures. The fundamental question asked was, if teeth are to be restored with a material of physical properties inferior to those of enamel, should large amounts of tooth substance be removed during cavity preparation? The answer to this question is that as much tooth structure should be preserved as possible by preparing cavities which are only large enough to allow removal of all caries.

It is also now appreciated that dental caries is not a continuous process of demineralization, but attempts at repair occur at the same time, which may halt the advance of the lesion. If preventive methods are also used, such as dietary counselling, effective plaque removal and using fluoride dentifrices, then early enamel lesions may partially repair and the progression of other lesions may stop. Of course, caries not only attacks enamel but cementum and dentine, and as people now have a greater life expectancy, so dental health care workers will increasingly face the challenge of root caries. In this section enamel and dentine caries will be covered together with the development of root surface caries.

Causes of dental caries

Dental plaque develops on the tooth surface as the result of a progressive build-up of different microbial species which leads to the development of a microbial community. The composition of this community depends on two factors:

1. The ability of micro-organisms to colonize either the acquired pellicle (derived from saliva) covering enamel surfaces, or other micro-organisms that have previously been living on the tooth surface.
2. The ability of other micro-organisms to grow on the surface in competition with the other members of the community.

This can be explained more simply be imagining the very special characteristics of dental plaque which may favour the growth of certain types of bacteria at different times. In some situations one species may have such an advantage that it becomes the major micro-organism of the community. This is termed dominance of one microbial species over others. Once microbial dominance has been achieved then the pathogenic potential of that organism is more easily expressed. Without doubt the most significant group of micro-organisms associated with dental caries in the mouth are the *Streptococcus mutans* group. In addition, the *Lactobacillus* group of micro-organisms is also significant in the caries process. Microbial dominance may not be sufficient by itself to produce caries; environmental factors also play a part.

Hence, dental caries appears to be initiated by acid produced in dental plaque which then attacks tooth structure. This process is very complex and is influenced by two groups of host-associated factors classified as environmental and genetic. The role of dental plaque in caries is covered in more detail in Chapter 5.

Environmental factors
Environmental factors which may hasten carious attack include:

1. Oral hygiene status. If a large amount of plaque is present the chances of a carious lesion developing increases.
2. The components of the diet. In this case a high carbohydrate intake allows increased microbial activity in plaque and as a result the production of lactic and pyruvic acids.
3. Salivary flow rate. Reduced salivary flow allows plaque to accumulate more readily and when combined with the loss of the protective buffering action of saliva, caries development can be rapid.
4. Drug therapy. Many drugs can affect the mouth and antidepressants are a good example. They are commonly prescribed and often depress salivary flow.

Genetic factors
These include the following:

1. Tooth morphology and enamel mineral composition.
2. Overcrowding in the dental arch.

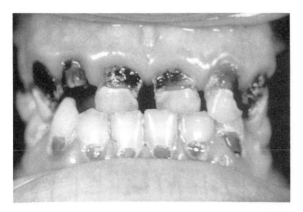

Figure 4.1   Marked cervical caries seen in a patient with a neglected mouth

3. Salivary composition including the presence of such antimicrobials as urea and lysozyme, and the availability of bicarbonate which affects buffering capacity.
4. Host immune defence mechanisms.

Types of caries

There are various types of caries which may be classified in two different ways. The first classification relates to the site of attack:

1. Enamel caries which can be subdivided into pit, fissure and smooth surface.
2. Root caries which develops following cemental exposure when gingival recession has occurred (Figure 4.1).
3. Recurrent caries which is seen at the margins or underneath an existing restoration (Figure 4.2).

The second classification is based on the rate of progression of the carious lesion:

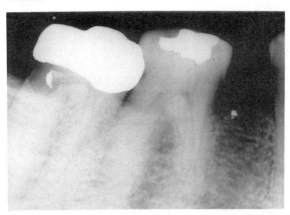

Figure 4.2   Recurrent caries visible beneath the distal margin of the crown on 47

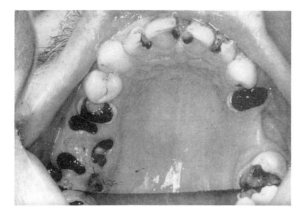

Figure 4.3   Acute or rampant caries in a young patient. This is now rarely seen due to the use of fluoridated dentifrices and improved oral hygiene practices

1. Acute (rampant) caries where there is rapid destruction of tooth tissue involving tooth surfaces that are normally considered to be fairly resistant to attack. It is seen in young patients (Figure 4.3).
2. Chronic (slowly progressive) caries. It is often seen in older patients and when it occurs in dentine allows time for secondary dentine formation.
3. Arrested caries occurs where enamel or dentine caries shows no tendency for progression.

Enamel caries

The first clinical indication that enamel has been damaged by acids produced in dental plaque is the presence of the 'white spot lesion'. These lesions form in areas where plaque collects, such as the pits and fissures of the occlusal surfaces, and on the smooth surfaces approximally where teeth contact each other, and also just above the gingival margin. The white spot represents a very early demineralization, but the enamel surface remains unbroken and is quite hard to probing. If this type of lesion has been present in the mouth for some time then it may be brown in colour and is naturally called a 'brown spot lesion'. The subsequent fate of these early white spot lesions is either remineralization following good plaque control or if plaque remains the enamel surface will further break down to form a cavity. To detect white or brown spot lesions the teeth need to be free of plaque, as dry as possible, and examined under a good light.

Microscopic appearance of enamel caries

Smooth surface caries
Under a microscope the smooth surface lesion is usually triangular in shape with the apex pointing towards the pulp chamber. The lesion consists of four zones which are apparent when a longitudinal section of tooth is viewed with a light microscope. There is a translucent zone which is present at the advancing front of the lesion, and a dark zone just behind this. The body of

the lesion forms the third zone with the apparently intact surface enamel forming the fourth zone.

Fissure caries
The pits and fissures on teeth are obvious points of plaque stagnation and because of their size deny access to toothbrush bristles. The histological appearance of fissure caries is similar to the smooth surface lesion. It starts in the enamel in each side wall of the fissure giving the appearance of two smooth surface lesions. Eventually, the two lesions join at the base of the fissure and the caries spreads both towards the pulp and laterally, taking on the shape of a triangle but this time the base is towards the pulp, while the apex points to the fissure.

Arrested enamel caries
These lesions are quite commonly seen on the cervical margins of teeth, where bands of demineralization have occurred just after eruption. As passive eruption takes place these bands become clear of the gingival margin and hence less prone to plaque collection. Other sites which may reveal such lesions are on the mesial or distal surfaces of posterior teeth when the adjacent tooth has been extracted. The loss of the adjacent tooth allows more efficient plaque removal in a site that would normally only be cleansable by flossing. This arrest of the carious process may allow mineral to be redeposited within the lesion from saliva, a process termed remineralization.

Clinical detection of enamel caries
The diagnosis of caries requires good lighting together with dry and plaque-free teeth. The use of a sharp dental probe is not recommended as this may physically damage an early carious lesion; indeed a blunt probe is now considered to be the ideal explorer for examining pits and fissures. In addition, bitewing radiographs are useful to detect occlusal as well as approximal caries, although by the time the lesion is visible on a radiograph it has usually involved dentine. There are other ways of detecting caries and reference to a more detailed text is recommended for this information.

In the adult mouth it has been shown that dental caries is a very slow disease taking between 2 and 4 years to progress through the enamel. This observation prompted certain researchers to question the value of the 6-monthly dental check-up and created lively discussion amongst dentists. However, with the possibility for remineralization of the early lesion the opportunity for prescribing effective prevention arises and a 6-monthly examination would appear to be more attractive.

Dentine caries
When caries reaches the enamel/dentine junction it spreads laterally as well as in a pulpal direction. Caries in dentine is again triangular in shape but with the apex pointing towards the pulp. The caries process in dentine tends to spread very rapidly in deciduous teeth and recently erupted permanent teeth. This is due to the presence of large dentinal tubules which allow entry of micro-organisms into the substance of dentine. In recently erupted

permanent teeth dentinal tubules tend to be quite large and the band of peritubular dentine which surrounds the tubule is thin, and is therefore quite easily penetrated by cariogenic bacteria. Dentine caries in the older patient progresses at a slower rate because the dentine will have become more sclerotic with narrower dentinal tubules, providing a more effective barrier to bacterial invasion.

Root caries

This is thought to represent the new challenge in dentistry. Its incidence is rising now that people are living longer and retaining more teeth. Recent statistics indicate that in the UK by the year 2000 only 10% of the population will be edentulous compared with 37% in 1968. Therefore a greater proportion of the over 60s will keep their natural teeth. The clinical presentation of root caries reveals that both active and inactive (arrested) types of lesion can be identified. It is seen more commonly on the buccal and approximal surfaces of teeth. The active lesions are soft and yellow or light brown in colour, while the arrested lesions tend to be hard, shiny and more darkly stained.

Several active lesions can coalesce and may encircle the tooth but if the gingiva recedes further then a lesion may become inactive. Cavity formation is commonly seen in active lesions and thick yellow or white plaque often fills the defects. It is interesting to note that pain due to pulpal involvement is not very common. The diagnosis of root caries requires a plaque-free surface, sharp eyes and a blunt probe. As with enamel caries a sharp instrument will readily damage the softened root surface.

There are several factors which predispose to root caries. The exposure of cementum as a result of gingival recession is a prerequisite for this type of carious attack. Secondly, xerostomia or dry mouth favours the development of root caries and this condition is more common in the elderly as a result of drug therapy which may affect salivary flow rate, or a consequence of radiotherapy to the head and neck region (Figure 4.4). Dietary factors, particularly the consumption of frequent sugary drinks or sucking of sweets,

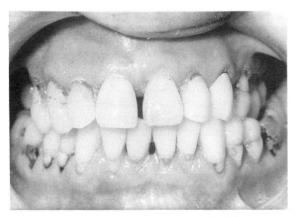

Figure 4.4   A patient suffering from xerostomia following radiation therapy for a malignancy of the neck. Extensive cervical restorations and new carious lesions.

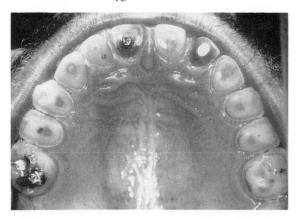

Figure 4.5   Tooth surface loss due to erosion in a patient who suffers from gastric acid reflux. The upper palatal surfaces are more affected than the buccal

will compromise the exposed root surface even more. The psychological pressures arising from retirement, ill health and bereavement may allow quite marked changes in diet to occur with an increased consumption of convenience foods being quite common. Finally elderly people find it more difficult to carry out effective tooth cleaning and indeed may not consider oral hygiene to be a priority.

Tooth surface loss

The use of the term 'tooth surface loss' has become popular in the last few years and it is used to describe tooth tissue loss due to erosion, attrition and abrasion. It does not replace these terms but is used before a definitive diagnosis can be made, usually at the patient's first visit.

Erosion

Erosion is the loss of enamel and dentine resulting primarily from attack by acid (Figure 4.5). If dietary or other acids are applied to the surface of an extracted tooth, etching occurs. This frosty white surface does not resemble the types of lesions that are seen in the mouth as result of erosion. This is because in the mouth there is a secondary factor involved which rubs away the softened decalcified surface to produce a smooth surface. The secondary factor is usually attrition by opposing teeth or abrasion by dietary factors. Erosion is almost always caused by acid from one of three sources: hydrochloric acid regurgitated from the stomach, acids from the diet, or from acid atmospheric pollution in the workplace. Regurgitation is not unusual in the elderly where chronic indigestion and hiatus hernia may be present, but it is also seen in anorexia nervosa and this may be the reason for abnormal tooth wear in a young person (Figure 4.6).

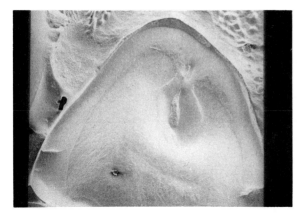

Figure 4.6   A scanning electron micrograph of a palatal tooth surface in a patient with bulimia. The selective 'sparing' of the gingival margin can be seen

Dental erosion may also be seen in older people suffering from dry mouth because the flow of saliva is much reduced. Patients who might at one time have eaten several items of fruit per day with no ill effects now suffer from erosion due to the loss of the protective functions of saliva. Chronic alcoholism may also allow regurgitation to occur although the individual may be unaware of it. The popular image of the chronic alcoholic being a derelict is true for a small minority who would very rarely seek dental treatment; the discreet middle class alcoholic is much more likely to seek dental advice for the problems of tooth wear.

Attrition

This is wear as a result of tooth-to-tooth contact. It may be seen if the diet has a very abrasive component or if the teeth are used as a tool which is common in Eskimo populations. It is commonly seen in developed countries when clenching or tooth grinding habits are taking place (Figure 4.7). These

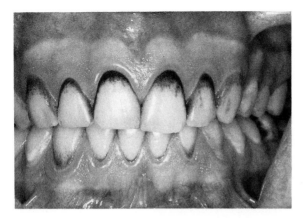

Figure 4.7   Attrition of the incisal edges of 13, 12, 11 while 21, 22, 23 are unaffected. There is also present a green extrinsic stain in the cervical area

habits are very complex in nature and 'bruxism' is a combination of dental, emotional, occupational and systemic factors. Attrition is commonly seen as wear facets which are small polished areas on enamel surfaces where heavy tooth contact is occurring. Once dentine is exposed, and especially if acid erosion is also present, then 'cupping' will occur as dentine is worn away more quickly.

Abrasion

This is the progressive loss of hard tooth substance caused by mechanical factors other than mastication or tooth-to-tooth contacts. Examples of this include destructive tooth brushing techniques and life-long habits such as pipe smoking (Figure 4.8) where the pipe is continually held in the mouth. Abrasion due to working in a dust polluted environment is less commonly seen now as a result of improved working conditions. Such conditions may still be found in coal mines or brick works and may be seen in employees who fail to wear protective masks.

Management of tooth wear

The management of a patient who presents with tooth wear has two phases. The first is to monitor the progression of wear using serial study models and clinical photographs and during this time take all steps possible to prevent further deterioration. Secondly, if the wear is found to be progressing to the extent that any further tissue loss is going to be difficult to restore, after careful treatment planning and, if possible, correction of aetiological factors, reconstruction of the worn dentition should be considered.

Enamel hypoplasia

This occurs when there is a defect in enamel matrix during tooth development and may be seen as a result of an hereditary condition, or due to

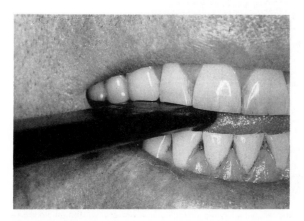

Figure 4.8 Abrasion due to pipe smoking

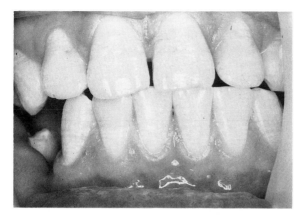

Figure 4.9 Amelogenesis imperfecta – showing ridged and discoloured enamel

constitutional disturbances during childhood. The best example of the first type is seen in amelogenesis imperfecta, which is an inherited condition of variable genetic penetrance affecting enamel and no other tissues of the body. The enamel is often pitted, coloured yellow or brown and in some severely affected cases absent (Figure 4.9). It is present in both dentitions.

The second type of enamel hypoplasia is caused by environmental factors and may only affect one tooth or several teeth in either dentition. It is known that several different factors which are each capable of disturbing ameloblast activity may give rise to the condition. The circumstances in which this type of hyperplasia can occur include:

1. Exanthematous disease (measles, chicken pox, etc. see Figure 4.10).
2. Apical abscess on a deciduous tooth.
3. Congenital syphilis (Hutchinson's incisors, Mulberry molars).
4. Chemical   imbalance   seen   in   excessive   fluoride   intake.

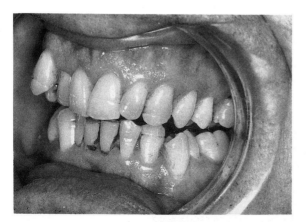

Figure 4.10 Chronological hyperplasia: a hypoplastic line can be seen on the incisors and canines

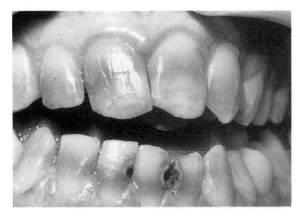

Figure 4.11   Tetracycline stained teeth showing typical dark discolouration. Two bands of staining are seen, a grey band in the middle of the crown and another yellow band near the gingival margin

Iatrogenic dental pathology

A dictionary defines iatrogenic as 'caused by medical examination or treatment'. Therefore, iatrogenically induced dental pathology relates to any dental disease which may develop as a result of treatment. Iatrogenic dental pathology can be conveniently grouped under two headings depending on whether systemic or local treatment has produced the problem. Systemically induced conditions include dental fluorosis and tetracycline staining.

In tetracycline staining of teeth, the antibiotic has to be administered to the patient, who is usually a child, while the teeth are developing (Figure 4.11). This condition is now infrequently seen as physicians are more aware of this side effect.

Enamel fluorosis can be produced by continuous low level exposure, multiple higher levels of exposure, or a single high fluoride dose. This could occur from drinking water with more than the optimum concentration of fluoride, or by use of a fluoride dentifrice (in a young child) and fluoride supplements (Figure 4.12). In mild fluorosis the tooth tends to lose its lustre

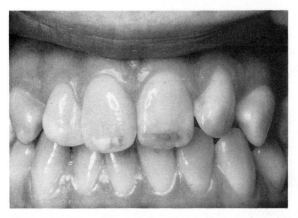

Figure 4.12   Enamel fluorosis involving the incisal edges of 11 and 21

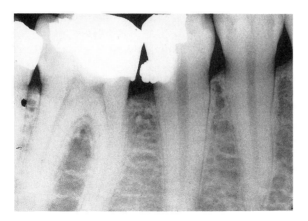

Figure 4.13 Amalgam overhangs on both 46 and 45 with early bone loss evident on the distal aspect of 45

and when its surface is dried, small white patches can be seen. The condition is rarely unsightly. More obvious mottling is characterized by yellow or brown stains in the enamel. In severe mottling the surface of the enamel is hypoplastic and will often appear very unsightly. This type of enamel fluorosis is still seen in people who live in developing countries and drink water from wells which contain fluoride levels in excess of 6 parts per million.

A commonly seen local example of iatrogenic pathology is where a restoration is placed, which is poorly contoured at the gingival margin, resulting in the presence of an overhang (Figure 4.13) with subsequent periodontal breakdown. A further commonly seen example is the gingival inflammation that can develop in relation to full crowns (Figure 4.14). Both of these conditions are the result of increased plaque retention due to the poor marginal contour of these types of restoration. The suggested way of preventing this type of problem is to place the margins of restorations, whenever possible, supragingivally.

In mouths which exhibit a considerable amount of restorative work,

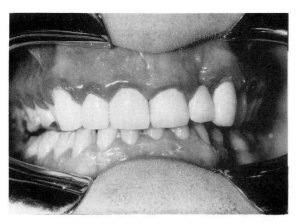

Figure 4.14 Typical gingival inflammation of a patient with poorly contoured, plaque retentive upper anterior crowns

plaque retention increases where restorations are in intimate contact with the gingival margin. Where good quality restorative work has been provided for a patient, its ultimate success is dependent on keeping plaque levels to a minimum. The contour of a crown at the gingival margin may have been distorted by shrinkage of the porcelain facing during its fabrication in the laboratory, hence a poor marginal adaptation is seen when the crown is placed.

Chapter 5

Dental deposits

Dental plaque

Dental plaque may be defined as bacterial aggregations on the teeth or other solid oral structures (Egelberg, 1970). This definition is not universally accepted, although for clinical purposes it is quite adequate and simple to remember. Plaque will form on tooth surfaces, restorations and oral appliances and the initial film which heralds the onset of plaque formation, the acquired pellicle, is deposited within minutes of a tooth surface being cleaned. When mature plaque is examined under a microscope, it can be seen to be composed of micro-organisms of various types together with desquamated oral epithelial cells, erythrocytes and polymorphonuclear leucocytes. Contrary to popular belief, dietary remains are rarely identified in plaque.

Two types of plaque are found at the gingival margin: supragingival which forms above the gingival margin and can be easily identified with disclosing solution, and subgingival which forms below the gingival margin and is always present on the root surfaces in periodontal pockets. Supragingival plaque is always deposited first.

Formation

The first stage in plaque formation is the laying down of acquired pellicle, which is derived from salivary glycoprotein and is actually a mucoprotein deposited on the tooth surface very soon after brushing. The acquired pellicle is initially devoid of micro-organisms but within 3–8 hours of its deposition streptococci begin to form colonies. Most of these have been identified as *Streptococcus mitis* and *Streptococcus sanguis* with *Streptococcus milleri* also being present but in smaller numbers. *Streptococcus mutans*, if present at this stage, only occurs in very low numbers. Gram-positive rods such as *Actinomyces viscosus*, *Actinomyces naeslundii* and *Actinomyces odontolyticus* may also be present in this early plaque. It is not until 24 hours have elapsed that this plaque will have become clinically evident. After the first 24 hours, changes in the proportions of micro-organisms take place. The proportion of streptococci decrease to about 45% while Gram-negative anaerobic cocci such as *Veillonella alcalescens* rapidly increase to around 20% of total organisms present. After 3 days the proportions of Gram-negative cocci and rods continue to increase and at 7 days a complex plaque flora will be present consisting of spirochaetes, fusiform bacilli, filamentous organisms and large numbers of Gram-negative cocci and bacilli. During the next 3 weeks of undisturbed plaque formation further changes occur as the bulk of plaque builds up to favour the growth of anaerobic organisms like Porphyromonas (*Bacteroides*) species. Plaque which is 3 weeks old will also reveal a significant number of non-viable micro-organisms (Figure 5.1).

Subgingival plaque forms from established supragingival plaque. However, the subgingival environment will influence the growth conditions of this area. The level of oxygen is low so favouring the growth of anaerobic bacteria. Nutrients for these organisms come from the crevicular fluid and the volume is increased as a result of the inflammation which is already present.

Micro-organisms which do not possess a special adhesion mechanism to plaque can survive in the protected environment of the developing pocket. Some of these factors may explain why the microbiology of subgingival plaque is different from the supragingival variety.

In patients who have suffered from gingivitis for 2–3 months, streptococci account for 25% of the total organisms present with *S. mitis* and *S. sanguis* being the most prolific. A further 25% is accounted for by *Actinomyces* species. Gram-negative anaerobic rods contribute a further 25% with *Fusobacteria*, Porphyromonas (*Bacteroides*), *Wolinella* and *Campylobacter* prominent. Spirochaetes are not readily cultured but they may account for 2% of plaque organisms in a patient exhibiting gingivitis (Figure 5.2).

In advanced periodontal disease with deep pockets the microbial population is different again. Here, 90% of the cultivable microbiota will be anaerobes. These anaerobic Gram-negative bacteria are mainly *Bacteroides* species and *Fusobacteria nucleatum*. Spirochaetes are very prominent in deep pockets accounting, in some instances, for up to 50% of micro-organisms present. In the specific form of periodontal disease termed juvenile periodontitis, the subgingival flora is different again. In this condition a

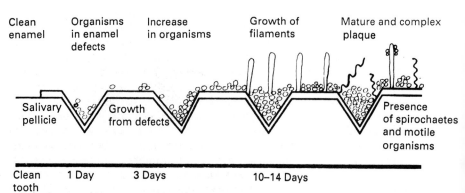

Figure 5.1 Diagrammatic representation of plaque maturation

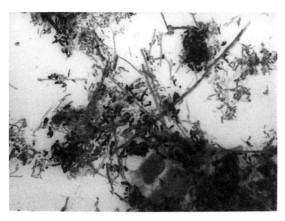

Figure 5.2   A smear of mature dental plaque showing dark staining Gram-positive cocci, light staining Gram-negative bacilli, with a single neutrophil in the lower part of the picture. The large 'fibres' are *Leptotricia*

Gram-negative rod, *Actinobacillus actinomycetemcomitans*, has been identified, with spirochaetes accounting for up to 7% of the total flora.

Structure of dental plaque

The first cellular material adhering to the pellicle on the tooth surface or other solid surface consists of coccal bacteria with small numbers of epithelial cells and polymorphonuclear leucocytes. Bacteria may be encountered within the pellicle as single organisms or as aggregates. After a few days various species will be present and it can be demonstrated that some benefit is derived from a symbiotic relationship with others; a good example of this is the 'corn on the cob' configuration which is seen at this stage where cocci grow on the surface of filamentous organisms. The material present between the bacteria is known as intermicrobial matrix and accounts for 25% of the plaque volume. Three sources may contribute to this matrix: plaque micro-organisms, saliva and gingival fluid.

Bacterial metabolism produces various end products. Some bacteria produce extracellular carbohydrate polymers which can act as an energy store or an anchoring material for micro-organisms in plaque. Dead bacteria will also contribute to the matrix. Different bacteria will have different metabolic pathways and therefore the matrix of plaque will vary considerably from one area to another. Several oral streptococci can synthesize fructans and glucans from dietary sucrose. The insoluble glucans are thought to play an important part in aggregating bacteria on the tooth surface whilst soluble fructans are utilized as a food source in bacterial metabolism. In parts of plaque where Gram-negative organisms are present, the intermicrobial substance contains small vesicles which have a similar structure to the outer cell wall of Gram-negative organisms. It is thought that these vesicles may contain lipopolysaccharides (endotoxins) and proteolytic enzymes. In subgingival plaque which is forming on the root surface, the structure appears to be similar to supragingival accumulations except that a large number of leucocytes are present. Where a deep pocket is present these leucocytes (which are predominantly neutrophils) are interposed between the gingival sulcular epithelium and the surface of the bacterial deposit and there is very little intermicrobial matrix.

Diet and plaque formation

Diet plays an important part in plaque formation, but two opposing factors may be operating. One is a diet which involves vigorous chewing which will stimulate the cleansing and buffering action of saliva, or the other which is a soft sugary diet which will encourage the formation of plaque. Experiments in dogs have shown that a hard fibrous diet reduces plaque formation. In man similar investigations when chewing apple or raw carrot have not produced the same result. The difference may be explained by the different dental anatomy in dogs compared with man. The teeth of dogs tend to be conical in shape and spaced which would allow a fibrous food to exert a more effective cleansing action than would be the case in the human mouth (Figure 5.3a and b).

Plaque and caries

The role of dental plaque in producing dental caries was first described by W. D. Miller in a series of research papers first published around the beginning of the 20th century. However, very little further research was carried out until the 1950s when Orland and Keyes showed that micro-organisms were essential in the development of the carious lesion. In 1960 Keyes in a very important research paper showed that when germ-free animals were infected with known strains of streptococci these bacteria could be transferred to uninfected animals who subsequently developed caries. Hence he demonstrated that dental caries was potentially infectious. In subsequent work using gnotobiotic rodents (animals infected with a known population of bacteria) it was found that the most important organisms for the production of caries were *Streptococcus mutans* and also some strains of lactobacilli and actinomycetes. Later work using monkeys infected with these organisms confirmed the importance of a high carbohydrate diet and also that a mother could transmit the disease to her offspring.

Streptococcus mutans and lactobacilli are able to produce caries because as they metabolize fermentable dietary carbohydrate they produce acid as a by-product. They are known as aciduric organisms because they thrive in acid conditions. In addition, they produce the extracellular polysaccharides, glucan and fructan, from the metabolism of sucrose, and these help to stick the organisms together as well as forming the matrix of plaque. This bulky plaque matrix is also very effective in preventing the buffering action of saliva, neutralizing the acid produced in plaque. Therefore, a greater plaque deposit means more acid production together with an increased barrier to saliva and the tooth surface will more easily demineralize.

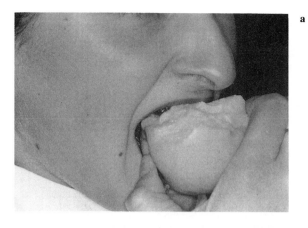

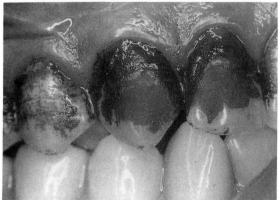

Figure 5.3   The effects of mastication on mature plaque: (a) volunteer chewing an apple after avoiding tooth brushing for 14 days; (b) the teeth disclosed after eating showing plaque deposits still present

Plaque and dietary carbohydrate

The importance of carbohydrates in the production of dental caries is well established but some aspects are more significant than others. For example, polysaccharides such as starch are mainly harmless as they are incompletely digested in the mouth. The monosaccharides and disaccharides (sugars) are considerably more important as they are readily broken down by bacteria in plaque to produce acid. The plaque will remain at a low level of acidity for a while, before returning to its more usual pH of 7. Therefore, frequent intakes of sugar-rich foods will keep plaque pH constantly below the critical level, resulting in demineralization of the tooth surface. For this reason, eating snacks between meals is discouraged because they are rich in carbohydrate which can be fermented by plaque bacteria, allowing the production of lactic acid which will in turn produce tooth surface demineralization.

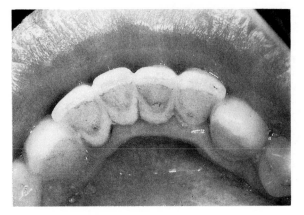

Figure 5.4   The appearance of supragingival calculus

Dental calculus

Dental calculus may be defined as the calcified or calcifying deposit on teeth or other solid structures present in the mouth. A dental prosthesis will often exhibit calculus formation if it is not kept clean, but calculus deposits on natural teeth are more common, when supragingival and subgingival deposit may be seen. The clinical appearance of supragingival calculus is of a yellow or white deposit on the tooth surface usually at the gingival margin (Figure 5.4). The colour may change to brown as a result of secondary staining from the use of tobacco or foodstuffs, particularly strong tea or coffee (Figure 5.5). The largest amounts of supragingival calculus appear opposite the openings of the major salivary glands on the buccal surfaces of maxillary molars and the lingual surfaces of lower incisors. By way of contrast, subgingival calculus is brown to black in colour, of a harder consistency and often more difficult to remove, and occurs on the roots of teeth with periodontal pocketing.

Diagnosis

Calculus when present supragingivally in reasonable amounts can be seen quite easily. However, when in thin section and moistened by saliva it can be easily missed so it is important to dry the tooth surface before exploring with an instrument. Subgingival calculus is considerably more difficult to detect although its position just below the gingival margin may produce a dark shadow in the marginal gingivae. In deeper pockets its presence can be detected by instruments such as a Cross calculus probe or by using a WHO type periodontal probe. Carefully directing air from a triple syringe into an active pocket will open the entrance to the pocket revealing the root surface on which calculus deposits may be evident. It may also be detected on radiographs where it can be seen as 'calculus spurs', most commonly at the junction of the crown and root. This method does not reveal the thin

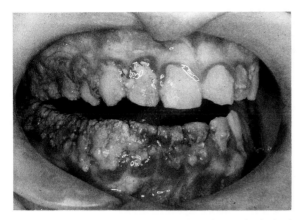

Figure 5.5   A more unusual presentation of supragingival calculus

deposits of plaque-like subgingival calculus that may form on teeth that have deep periodontal pockets and, of course, errors in radiographic technique or film development may mask the presence of calculus. Therefore the best means of detection is by palpation.

Composition and structure of calculus

Calculus consists of 70–80% inorganic material of which approximately 60% is in crystalline form. The four principal crystal forms are hydroxyapatite, whitlockite, brushite and octacalcium phosphate. Brushite tends to be more common in supragingival calculus, whilst whitlockite is found particularly in subgingival calculus. The organic component of calculus consists predominantly of proteins and carbohydrates with lipids accounting for only a very small proportion.

The structure of calculus has proved difficult to investigate due to its high mineral content, but with the use of the electron microscope and the ability to cut it into ultra-thin sections a clear picture has emerged. Ground sections of calculus have revealed it to have a layered structure and the level of calcification can vary between the layers. The crystals are randomly arranged although areas can be found in which the crystals are all lying in the same direction but these areas are uncommon. A significant finding in the structure of calculus is that it always exhibits a layer of unmineralized plaque on its surface.

Formation of calculus

Calculus formation is always preceded by plaque formation which provides the organic matrix in which mineralization can occur. Initially, crystals can be seen to form in the intermicrobial matrix of plaque, commonly in close apposition to bacteria. The number of crystals rises with the passage of time, until eventually the bacteria themselves also become mineralized. Several hypotheses have been proposed for the appearance of these crystals in dental plaque which heralds calculus formation.

The carbon dioxide hypothesis is one which states that the level of CO_2 present in saliva which leaves the ducts of the salivary glands is considerably higher than that found in the saliva in the mouth. This difference will result in the escape of CO_2 from saliva producing a rise in pH. When the pH of saliva rises it can hold less calcium and phosphate ions in solution, hence spontaneous precipitation occurs. Once crystals have developed they will stimulate the formation of others until the level of mineralization seen in calculus is reached. This theory may explain why supragingival calculus develops near the openings of the major salivary gland ducts, but it does not explain how subgingival calculus may form.

Another hypothesis states that ammonia production produces a rise in plaque pH because it has been shown that rapid calculus formers have an increased urea concentration in their saliva. Ammonia is a breakdown product of urea and the breakdown of proteins in plaque might result in the local production of urea and ammonia, hence a local increase in the pH of plaque which would induce the local precipitation of calcium and phosphate ions.

The nucleation theory is another proposal for the development of calculus. When crystallization is nucleated (started) by a compound of different chemical composition, in this case the organic matrix of plaque, the phenomenon is termed epitaxis. However, the compound(s) which may be responsible for nucleation in plaque has yet to be identified.

Micro-organisms which are degenerating under experimental conditions have been shown to form calcium phosphate crystals of the same type as those seen in calculus. Recent research has identified a protease enzyme isolated from *Bacteroides loeschii* which is common in plaque and may affect the properties of saliva which would result in the precipitation of calcium and phosphate ions. It would seem reasonable to assign a key role for the initiation of crystal formation in plaque to the bacteria present, but this does not mean that they alone are responsible for the production of possible nucleating compounds. Indeed, calculus has been shown to occur in germ-free rats, albeit in small quantities, where it is thought to be due to the deposition and calcification of organic matrix from saliva.

Attachment of calculus to the tooth surface

Calculus often adheres to teeth tenaciously and the removal of subgingival calculus can be especially difficult. One of the reasons for this strong attachment may be that the pellicle beneath the plaque also calcifies and hence calculus crystals come into intimate contact with those found in cementum, enamel or dentine. Furthermore, the tooth surface irregularities are penetrated by calculus crystals so that the calculus becomes virtually locked onto the tooth surface. On the surface of cementum this is particularly the case since the spaces once occupied by the Sharpey's fibres in the periodontal ligament leave small pits in which calculus crystals may grow. As a result, it is impossible to remove all calculus from the surface of the tooth without the loss of a small amount of tooth tissue.

Significance of calculus

Calculus is invariably associated with periodontal disease as it is always covered with plaque. It is difficult to confirm whether calculus would produce any detrimental effects if there were no plaque present. Recently it has been proposed that, provided the surface of calculus can be rendered smooth by polishing, its potential to retain plaque is much reduced. This confirms research conducted a few years ago which revealed that under certain circumstances a normal attachment may be seen between junctional epithelium and calculus.

The main role of calculus in the initiation of periodontal disease would appear to be as a site to retain plaque. Its presence may hamper efficient plaque removal procedures by the patient and it may act as a reservoir for the toxic by-products of plaque metabolism in periodontal pockets. Also the presence of excessive amounts of calculus may inhibit the drainage of inflammatory products from periodontal pockets and as a consequence increase the possibility of a periodontal abscess. It is not the most important factor in the initiation of periodontal disease but it may be described as an aggravating factor in disease progression.

Stains on teeth

Stains on teeth are discolourations which may be extrinsic (occurring on the external surface) or intrinsic (in the tooth structure). Extrinsic stains can be removed by scaling and polishing or in some cases by more effective tooth brushing. A list of the commonly seen extrinsic and intrinsic stains can be seen in Table 5.1.

Table 5.1   Extrinsic stains which may be seen on teeth

Stain	Appearance	Development	Occurrence
Brown	Seen around necks of teeth	From tobacco usage	Smokers
Brown	Seen around necks of teeth and interproximally	From chlorhexidine mouthrinsing	When used for longer than 3 weeks.
Yellow	Dull yellow with whole of crown covered	From food pigments	Seen in all ages due to poor oral hygiene
Green	Green line around necks of teeth	? Chromogenic bacteria ? From blood pigment (via gingival bleeding)	Poor oral hygiene, often seen in children
Black	Black line around necks of teeth	Due to bacteria (Gram-positive rods)	All ages: often seen in females on maxillary molars; usually good oral hygiene present

Drinking large amounts of coffee and tea will leave a stain on teeth which is brown in colour. Some metals cause tooth staining, e.g. brass and copper produce a green stain and iron leaves a black stain. The source of the metals may be from the working environment and it is worthwhile asking about employment when such stains are seen.

Intrinsic stains may be caused by drugs such as tetracycline which, if taken during tooth development, will be incorporated into the dentine staining it grey-yellow. Corrosion products of dental amalgam may stain the tooth grey and the presence of dental caries will produce a stain, whether an active or inactive lesion. A non-vital tooth will often exhibit intrinsic staining if pulpal degeneration occurred before endodontic therapy was undertaken. The rare conditions of amelogenesis imperfecta and dentinogenesis imperfecta will produce staining and in severe cases of enamel fluorosis staining is present. Techniques are available which can treat or at least mask intrinsic staining but reference to another text is recommended for details of the methods available.

Part Three   Clinical Practice

Chapter 6

Patient assessment

It is vital that all dental personnel involved in patient care are able to make an accurate assessment of their patients, whether they carry the ultimate responsibility for their welfare or are under the direction of another member of the team. The assessment begins as patients enter the clinical area and their general appearance is registered, noting such factors as apprehension, unusual pallor, breathlessness, any visible handicap, and the general level of personal hygiene. The experienced clinician notes these factors automatically because they may indicate which types of treatment may be more acceptable. Apart from their names, patients' addresses and occupations are recorded. Both are factors which can indicate the amount of time available for treatment in terms of travelling time and 'time off work'. Treatment schedules can then be revised accordingly.

History

The patient's main complaint is considered first and in the case of periodontal disease could be bleeding gums, a bad taste, halitosis, drifting or loosening teeth, a gingival swelling, etc. It is best at this stage to let the patient describe the condition in his/her own words. Information is not always provided in a logical or concise manner and a degree of prompting may be needed by asking specific questions which could include: What is the problem? Which part of the mouth is affected? What makes it worse? How long have you had it?

Details of the dental history are recorded next and include information on attendance patterns, previous experience of local anaesthesia and if any ill effects from dental treatment have been experienced. Some take this opportunity to question home dental care practices such as brushing techniques and the use of floss but others believe this to be of little value as only an examination of the mouth will reveal the effectiveness of home care.

The medical history forms an important part of the information recorded. It is not only essential to record it at the first visit but to update it at each major recall appointment. This is particularly true as people grow older because the need for medical supervision tends to increase with age. The specific questions to ask when recording the medical history include the following:

1. Are you fit and healthy at present?
2. Have you had rheumatic fever or is there a history of heart disease?
3. Do you suffer from chest problems (bronchitis, emphysema, etc).
4. Are you allergic or hypersensitive to anything, especially drugs such as penicillin?
5. Are you taking medication from your doctor at present?
6. Have you ever suffered from hepatitis?
7. Is there any possibility that you may be HIV positive?
8. Do you suffer from diabetes mellitus?
9. Have you been admitted to hospital for any reason?
10. Do you bleed or bruise easily?
11. For women of childbearing age, enquire if they could be pregnant.

If there is a positive answer to any of the questions after the first, then further details may be required. It is important to include such details as the taking of the oral contraceptive pill. In some women the contraceptive pill may be associated with a low grade gingivitis, but more importantly its efficiency can be reduced by some broad-spectrum antibiotics, with the consequence of an unexpected pregnancy! At subsequent major recall visits there is no need to check every stage of the history again, but to check that it remains the same and specifically enquire about possible allergies that might have developed and any current medication.

Some clinicians now ask all new patients to complete a form which details their medical history and is signed by the patient. The advantage of this is to provide a patient-completed record of medical status which may be of use if medicolegal disputes arise. In some systemic diseases, further details may be required from the patient's physician (Table 6.1).

The social history is of some significance and details of tobacco use and alcohol consumption should be noted. The reason for inquiring into social

Table 6.1 An example of a simple medical history question-
naire that a patient could complete prior to seeing the clinician

MEDICAL HISTORY

HAVE YOU EVER HAD:

Rheumatic fever	YES/NO
Heart disease	YES/NO
Lung/chest disease	YES/NO
Bleeding problem	YES/NO
Allergy	YES/NO
Hepatitis	YES/NO
Blood transfusion	YES/NO
A serious operation	YES/NO
A serious illness	YES/NO
Are you taking any medicines	YES/NO

IF THE ANSWER TO ANY OF THESE QUESTIONS IS
YES, PLEASE DISCUSS WITH YOUR DENTIST

activities is that it will reflect the individual's attitude to health care and the prevention of disease. In addition, some chronic alcoholics may show evidence of dental erosion.

Clinical examination

Although a methodical clinical examination should be carried out by the dentist, other clinical staff such as hygienists should also be competent to undertake an examination of the mouth and related areas and recognize abnormal conditions. Prior to looking in the mouth, the condition of the lips is first noted especially for signs of herpes labialis, angular cheilosis, or general lip drying which may make the intraoral examination more difficult. Lip incompetence is also noted, as this can allow gingival drying to occur, which exacerbates the gingival reaction to plaque.

The oral mucosa must be examined and all of the lining mucosa evaluated. The lips, cheeks, vestibule, palate, dorsum of tongue, ventral surface of tongue and floor of mouth are all screened. Abnormalities such as ulcers or swellings, signs of infection, or mucosa which exhibits a change in colour, are noted. Some conditions, particularly white patches, can be asymptomatic and their presence is only detected by the vigilant clinician.

The teeth are next examined for caries. Restorations and cavities are charted and the quality of the restorations noted. Malaligned teeth should also be recorded in addition to those that demonstrate tooth wear because this may indicate a destructive toothbrushing habit or excessive occlusal loading. The level of oral hygiene is scored and the presence of plaque noted followed by the detection of supra- and subgingival calculus. This may be achieved using a Cross calculus probe for tactile detection or blowing air from the triple syringe into the pocket so allowing subgingival calculus to be seen. Where possible, plaque should be disclosed and shown to the patient.

The quality of gingival tissue is evaluated by noting the colour, contour and consistency of the gingiva whilst remembering it should be pink in colour (in the Caucasian subject) knife-edged to the tooth and well stippled and firm. The commoner signs and symptoms of inflammatory periodontal disease are shown in Table 6.2. Any degree of pathology may be encountered such as a periodontal abscess illustrated in Figure 6.1.

Pocket assessment

Pocket assessment should be undertaken using a graduated probe. There are a variety of probes available for this purpose and the choice is dependent on the individual clinician. The essence of periodontal pocket assessment is to record loss of periodontal attachment and ideally this should involve probing the gingival crevice at three points on the buccal and three points on the lingual surface as described in Chapter 12.

The probe must be inserted into the pocket as parallel to the tooth surface as possible and gently manipulated to avoid a false reading or patient

Table 6.2   The symptoms and signs that may be noted by a patient suffering from inflammatory periodontal disease

Symptoms	*Signs*
Bleeding gums	Gingiva
On brushing	*Red*
When eating	*Swollen*
Spontaneously	Teeth
	Mobile
Swollen gums	*Drifted*
Halitosis	Pockets
Loose teeth	*Deepened*
Moving teeth	*Pus*
Discharge from gums	*Bleeding on probing*
	Radiographs
	Bone loss
	Loss of lamina dura

discomfort. If there is considerable deposit present or the tissues are very inflamed, it may be better to delay pocket assessment until some of the deposit has been removed which will also allow some resolution of inflammation. Recording pocket depths is covered in the Appendix.

Tooth mobility

This is graded on a scale from 0 to 3; a score of 3 is allocated when the tooth can be moved up to 2 mm in any direction or depressed in its socket and generally indicates a tooth with a poor prognosis. This mobility scale is described in the Appendix.

Occlusion

The subject of occlusion is complex and is not within the remit of this book.

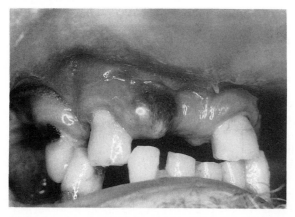

Figure 6.1   A periodontal abscess pointing on the mesial surface of 13

Nevertheless, an evaluation of the occlusal surfaces of the teeth is worthwhile, particularly when teeth are mobile or when an isolated area of gingival recession is identified which may indicate an increased clinical loading on that tooth. The use of study casts to examine occlusion more carefully is sometimes required. Abnormal cuspal contacts can be identified and corrected, particularly if an adjustable articulator is used in the occlusal analysis.

Special tests

The most common special tests employed to assist in diagnosis are radiographs. When, after the pocket assessment, a considerable loss of attachment is revealed, a decision must be made as to which films will be most useful. Most commonly, bitewing films of posterior teeth together with periapical films of the anteriors will illustrate the pattern of bone involvement. An orthopantomograph (OPG or OPT) will reveal the general pattern of bone involvement, but occasionally a full mouth radiographic examination is required and the paralleling technique should be used to avoid distortion (see Chapter 12).

In some patients the pattern of disease is such that a systemic condition may be suspected. In such cases more careful questioning of the patient about their general health together with any change in body function which has become apparent will point to a possible underlying cause. Special tests under these circumstances would include blood and possibly urine analysis together with any further investigations which are thought to be appropriate. Where a systemic condition is discovered then communication with the patient's physician is essential before providing any treatment.

A biopsy may be required to confirm the diagnosis if a localized gingival condition is apparent. Depending on the provisional diagnosis it may be worthwhile communicating with the histopathologist to enquire if the tissue should be sent in a particular way to allow, for example, immunological techniques to be used.

Assessment of prognosis

The response of disease to treatment is difficult to assess accurately, but before a definitive treatment plan can be devised a provisional assessment must be made, because in the case of periodontal disease, successful treatment is dependent on good cooperation from the patient in maintaining a high standard of plaque control. This is difficult to predict initially and so a provisional treatment plan should be given to the patient for consideration, while they undergo an initial plaque control programme involving regular review of their 'home care' on a weekly basis. If plaque levels are still too high after a 3-week period, motivation may be suspect and it would be worthwhile indicating your concern. Most research indicates that at best only 50% of patients will comply with regular brushing and flossing procedures and, of those who will not comply with professional advice, 70% will have given up totally before 3 months have elapsed. Hence, in the case of plaque control it is best to complete deposit removal professionally and instruct in home care, with a review appointment 3 months after the last attendance when resolution of inflammation (assuming good plaque control) should be maximal. If complicated periodontal treatment is required, a definitive treatment plan can now be formulated by the clinician in charge of the case.

The treatment plan

The treatment plan is devised to achieve three basic objectives, namely, to eradicate disease, to ensure restoration of function and to provide an acceptable appearance. It is important to remember that a degree of flexibility should be allowed in the treatment plan, particularly when dealing with periodontal disease, because the response of the tissues to treatment might not be as expected, particularly, for example, if the patient has refractory periodontitis.

Nutritional counselling

If the patient exhibits a high caries susceptibility, then the first point in the treatment plan, after carrying out any emergency care, would be to provide nutritional counselling after a 4-day diet diary has been completed. The object of this is to identify any obvious dietary factor increasing the caries rate. A typical diary is shown in Table 6.3 and is designed to include 2 week days and a weekend. The reason for including a weekend is because eating routines will be different from those of a week day. Patients should be told that all food and drink consumed on each day must be recorded, especially any intermeal snacks, so it is important to have the diary with them at all times. Also included should be the times that any drug therapy is administered. When the sheet is returned it should not be discussed with the patient at that visit. Time is needed for its careful evaluation and so it is discussed with the patient at the third visit. Nutritional counselling is a role that can be undertaken by the correctly trained and motivated dental assistant, or a dental health educator, or the dental hygienist.

When discussing the diet diary with the patient, the main points to consider are as follows:

1. Are the main meals substantial enough to make snacks unnecessary and is their nutritional value sufficiently high?
2. If intermeal snacks are listed, are they cariogenic?
3. The number and type of intermeal drinks, e.g. older patients with xerostomia may drink a lot of sweetened fruit juice between meals in the belief that this is beneficial.
4. Is sweet or candy consumption high?
5. Is any regular medication sucrose syrup-based?

Table 6.3   Diet Diary

Meal	Time	Type of food or drink	Approximate amount
Early morning			
Breakfast			
During morning			
Lunch			
During afternoon			
Tea			
Until bedtime			
During the night			

TIMES OF TOOTH CLEANING: . . . .

DAY . . . .   DATE . . . .

Ways of recording food and drink

Food	Examples	Approximate amount
Bread/toast/roll	White, wholemeal	Small/large slices Number
Cereal	Cornflakes/Frosties	Bowls
Biscuits	Plain/chocolate/sweet	Number
Cakes	Fruit/sponge	Number/slices
Puddings	Rice/crumble/custard	Bowls/portions of
Savoury snacks	Crisps/peanuts	Packets
Ice cream Ice lollies		Number
Sugar	When used in addition	Number of teaspoons
Meat/fish Eggs/Cheese	Types eg: fishfingers	Number or amount
Potatoes	Boiled/fried	Number or amount
Vegetables	Carrots/salad	Teaspoons or tablespoons
Fruit	Apple/peach/oranges	Number
Butter Margarine	If used	Teaspoons
Milk	Full cream semi-skimmed skimmed	Mug/cup/glass
Tea Coffee Chocolate	With or without sugar	
Fruit juice Squash	Type Type	
Lemonade	Sugar containing Low calorie	

6. Are any sweetened drinks taken before retiring to bed or kept by the bedside?

The diet diary should be kept in the patient's notes together with a record of the advice given.

Chapter 7

Patient management

One of the most radical changes to have occurred in dental teaching over the past ten years is the switch from an emphasis on instruction in technical skills to a recognition of the need for good diagnostic and management abilities. Even more recently the importance of interpersonal skills has been realized, not only to reinforce the concept of a dental health team, but also in ensure constructive clinician–patient relationships. Without these skills, effective communication with the patient, which provides the foundation for diagnostic and treatment decisions, cannot be established. Many of the advanced and complex restorative procedures now undertaken on patients are liable to ultimate failure, not because of technical problems, but because effective communication with the patient has not been developed.

Interpersonal relationships

There are a variety of differing relationships that may develop between dental health professionals and patients. The first, and most frequently observed relationship, is an 'active-passive' model in which the operator decides and undertakes the treatment with little or no patient involvement in decision making. Often when the problem is limited and the treatment choice clear, this type of relationship is sufficient, for example when minor scaling is the only therapy required. A variation on this approach is 'guidance-cooperation' where the patient is informed of the required action and then cooperates by following this advice. For simple dental health education, such as the need to undertake regular interdental cleaning, this role model should be appropriate. For more complex problems 'consensus-action' may be needed. This relationship may be applicable when complex problems exist and several treatment options are available. The final decision can only be made after considerable discussion between the patient and clinician. To arrive at this consensus requires a patient-centred approach using counselling techniques where the problem and possible outcomes are discussed fully with the patient who then makes an informed choice of the actions to be taken.

Barriers to communication

Many barriers to effective communication may exist between the operator and the patient. These may operate individually or in concert, and their importance will vary from patient to patient. The more important barriers are discussed below.

Social class and status

Differences in social class and status may constitute a barrier from both sides of the treatment divide. The clinician may be influenced for better or worse by the socioeconomic status of the patient. Patients of a lower class than the clinician may be regarded as unimportant or undeserving, with negative decisions being made as to the prognosis of teeth. For example, a periodontally involved tooth may be extracted when it could have been saved or at least retained for a further length of time. On the other hand the patient of a higher class may be over-treated for a similar problem, because the clinician may be reluctant to admit that the position is hopeless. Patients of a lower class may be reluctant to ask questions or ask for a different treatment and may be indifferent to treatment decisions, whereas higher class patients may not be prepared to value advice they receive from operators they perceive as belonging to a lower class than themselves.

Failure of comprehension

Patients who lack knowledge of their teeth or dental diseases may not be able to understand the importance of any advice given. The language used in explanations may contain a large amount of dental jargon, may be given at too great a speed and, in addition, the surrounding environment may cause difficulties in comprehension and inadequate recall. Research shows that patients are often unable to recall more than half of the advice given 5 minutes after the appointment has ended.

Cultural/ethnic differences

These may constitute significant barriers which are becoming more important as our 'global village' becomes more crowded and multi-cultural. As well as the problems of communicating effectively in a foreign language there may be other problems such as those groups which find tooth loss unacceptable for any reason. Some societies have strict chauvinistic beliefs which can make reasoned male/female communication difficult.

Fear and anxiety

Many patients attending for dental treatment may suffer from mild anxiety, whilst in a small minority this anxiety may be of such a level as to constitute actual fear. At its worst this may prevent the patient from attending for dental treatment but in those who do 'pluck up' courage to visit the surgery it may constitute a barrier to communication. For this reason it is important to establish successful communication before the clinical dental examination.

Interview and counselling techniques

Acquisition of the appropriate behaviour required to control established inflammatory periodontal disease needs considerable commitment by the patient, as the home care practices are both time consuming and tedious. Encouraging patients to make this commitment is one of the main aims of the interview and counselling process, as well as establishing the needs and expectations of the patient from any treatment.

The counselling process can be considered to have five phases, namely communication, assessment, understanding, treatment and maintenance.

Communication phase

In this phase the operator should identify the patients' complaints and clarify their attitudes towards the problem as well as assessing their knowledge and previous efforts at controlling the problem. It is useful to divide this phase into two, part of which is carried out before the assessment and the second completed after full information on the disease has been obtained. The communication phase should be aimed at helping the patient to recognize that a problem exists and establishing a desire to tackle the problem. This is not achieved by provision of technical information but by discussing the problem and possible solutions with the patient. It is best to conduct the initial interview with the patient away from the dental chair with all its intimidating equipment, preferably in a consulting room with as welcoming an atmosphere as possible. Furnishings such as soft lighting and fitted carpets are important together with easy chairs which may be side by side at a table or desk. The attitude of the operator should be sympathetic and non-threatening and the patient should not feel inhibited from asking questions or putting their point of view. Any opinions made by the patient should not be challenged directly but accepted with sympathy and understanding. All questions should be answered honestly without making negative judgements.

Assessment phase

This phase has two aims. The first is to establish the nature and extent of the disease and the second to assist in the communication phase by providing specific information. The assessment should include hard and soft tissue examination, the taking of suitable radiographs and, where appropriate, the making of study casts. The soft tissue examination should include the extraoral tissues and a detailed intraoral examination which should contain the following:

1. Mucosal health, including tongue, palate, cheeks and floor of mouth.
2. Gingival condition, preferably using an appropriate index, e.g. the bleeding index or gingival index.
3. Probing depths.
4. Plaque deposits, preferably using a plaque index.
5. Extent, position and type of calculus deposits.

The use of a treatment-needs index such as the Community Periodontal Index of Treatment Needs (CPITN) is considered by many periodontists to be an acceptable substitute for some of the above indices during the initial screening examination.

The hard tissue examination should also include:

1. Tooth mobility.
2. Existing restorations including their size and condition.
3. New cavities.

Wherever possible the investigation and its significance should be explained to the patient *before* the examination, which will enable the patient to understand the extent of the problem. If feasible the use of hand mirrors will allow them to watch the examination and enhance motivation.

Understanding phase

Once the patient has been examined and accepts the presence of disease and the need for its treatment, the understanding phase begins. It commences at the end of the assessment phase when the results of the examination are shown to the patient and the significance discussed. These results should also be given to the patient in the form of a simple written report. This is followed by the provision of information on how to treat the disease, with emphasis on the patient's role and responsibilities. The difficulties of treatment and home care measures should be frankly discussed but the patient given hope of mastering them. The time element in any treatment programme should be fully discussed with the patient.

Treatment phase

This phase has two closely related components. The patient component consists of learning more effective home care measures. Realistic goals for this should be agreed jointly. For example, it may be decided to increase the regularity of interdental cleaning from occasionally to daily. These goals or targets may be changed and increased with the patient's consent as the initial ones are attained, until optimal oral hygiene is achieved.

The operator component of the treatment phase consists of careful removal of root surface deposits, correction of any faulty restorations or prostheses, monitoring of the patient's progress and providing feedback. This treatment may take a considerable time and this should have been made clear to the patient during the understanding phase. During the time devoted to this treatment the patient's home care measures can be checked, improvements suggested and encouragement provided. The use of indices as described later will greatly assist this process.

Maintenance phase

Once the necessary level of home care has been achieved and the mouth has returned to health, the maintenance phase can commence. The essential elements of a maintenance programme are:

1. Monitoring the patient's condition to spot any deterioration.
2. Providing feedback and encouragement.
3. Providing further treatment to any areas showing recurrent breakdown.
4. Gradually increasing the period between reviews and thus encouraging the patient to take more responsibility for his/her own health.

Dental health education

The ultimate control of plaque-induced disease depends on patient oral hygiene habits which the clinician may find very difficult to alter, so subject are they to personal motivation. The anxious patient who has been sitting in the waiting room listening to the noises of the dental equipment, may not be initially receptive to oral hygiene advice until put at ease in the clinical environment. Indeed, a room set aside to provide oral health care advice is to be recommended, so that possible unpleasant memories of clinical dental practice are not recalled. When the patient is relaxed then the difficult task of stimulating motivation can begin. The approach to handling patients may be summarized as follows:

1. Meet the patient at an intellectual level appropriate to their education and background.
2. Indicate the benefits of prevention.
3. Set targets consisting of short-term goals to reduce disclosed plaque levels.
4. Comment favourably on any clinical improvements at follow-up.
5. Base any information given on currently acceptable scientific knowledge.

Home care technique

Dental health care workers are often asked how frequently teeth should be brushed. The answer would appear to be that for most people twice daily is adequate to maintain dental health, but for those suffering from dental disease more frequent brushing is indicated until gingival inflammation is resolved. Even ignoring the problem of the interproximal area, brushing twice daily can leave areas in the mouth that are consistently missed. Hence it is advisable to ask patients to concentrate on brushing very carefully on one occasion, such as the evening session, to thoroughly disrupt the plaque deposits that may occur in the more inaccessible areas.

The method of brushing is not critical provided that clinical plaque deposits are efficiently removed. Many patients will have developed their own techniques which may require only slight modification to achieve adequate plaque control and, provided that their brushing is not destructive in any way, then this is quite acceptable. Advice on brushing should always follow examination of the mouth and should relate to specific problems. Most patients are unaware of how tenacious dental plaque deposits are and this is often compounded by lack of understanding of dental anatomy. A further difficulty is that the average time taken to brush teeth is often no longer than 30 seconds, which is totally unsatisfactory even for the individual with a reasonable degree of manual dexterity. Ultimately, efficient plaque removal may depend on the time taken to brush away the deposits rather than the technique adopted.

Choice of toothbrush

Available toothbrushes vary considerably in their size, shape, bristle stiffness and tuft arrangement and this reflects the fact that there is no ideal specification that will permit efficient plaque removal in all subjects. Each patient will have an individual requirement. However, there is a general consensus among periodontists that the following general description would suit the average adult patient:

Size: 1.5–2.5 cm long and 0.15–0.75 cm wide.

Bristles: 2–4 rows, with 5–12 tufts in each row. The angulation of the tufts is not considered critical although many experts advocate a flat head for the brush.

Filaments: medium or soft nylon filaments are recommended by many, with a diameter that varies from 0.28 to 0.18 mm, although some studies have found that the more efficient plaque removal obtained with the larger diameters may be accompanied by gingival trauma. 6/10 nylon is frequently used with a 10–12 mm filament length. Suitable brushes are shown in Figure 7.1.

Specifically modified brushes are sometimes required for patients with mental or physical handicaps. These may have handles modified with autopolymerizing acrylic resin, arblaster paper or have a rubber collar placed over the handle (Figure 7.2). Electric toothbrushes, which generally are no more efficient than hand brushes, may have a role to play in these patients.

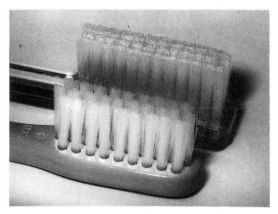

Figure 7.1   Suitable toothbrushes, with small heads and multitufted synthetic bristles

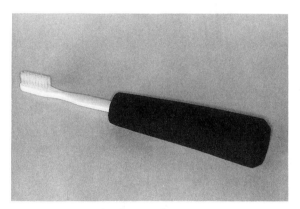

Figure 7.2   A toothbrush adapted for a patient with limited manual dexterity. The handle has been modified with a rubber collar which improves the ease of grip

Techniques of brushing

A variety of brushing techniques have been described which basically relate to the movement of the toothbrush head. These consist of:

1. Vibratory, e.g. Stillman, Charters, Bass.
2. Horizontal, e.g. Scrub, Miniscrub.
3. Roll, e.g. Rolling stroke, modified Stillman.
4. Circular, e.g. Fones.
5. Vertical, e.g. Physiological, Leonard.

Many patients attending the surgery will have been advised to use the Roll technique, as this was the favoured method in the 1970s. However recent evidence has suggested that this is an inefficient method. Although no one method of brushing has been shown to be superior to any other, as this will vary from patient to patient, the Bass and short scrub methods have been popular for a number of years and both these methods will be described.

The Miniscrub method

A variety of this technique – most correctly called a long scrub method – is the one adopted naturally by uninstructed patients and it is this fact that makes it most useful for adapting as part of efficient home care (Figure 7.3a).

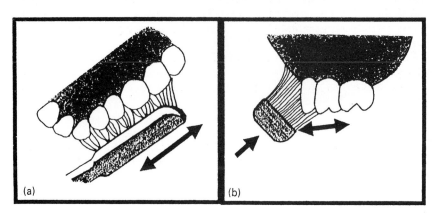

Figure 7.3 Methods of toothbrushing: (a) the Miniscrub method of toothbrushing. The bristles are placed at 90° to the tooth surface and moved back and forth with a small vibratory action. Limited subgingival penetration may occur; (b) the Bass method of toothbrushing. The bristles are placed at 45° to the tooth surface and moved back and forth with a small vibratory action. Subgingival penetration up to 3 mm can occur

A potential for damage occurs, however, when the bristles are dragged across the necks of the teeth causing abrasion. This problem may be avoided firstly by changing the grip on the handle from a palm to a finger grasp. Secondly, emphasis must be given to the activation, which should be a short vibratory action not a long horizontal scrub.

As well as being a simple, easily mastered method, the short scrub has the other advantage of permitting a limited amount of subgingival penetration, thus allowing pocket cleansing similar to that achieved with the Bass method.

Advantages
It is an easily learned, simple technique which requires minimal manual dexterity. The method cleans the gingival margin and penetrates subgingivally.

Disadvantages
Too aggressive an action may cause gingival recession and contribute to abrasion.

The Bass method

The aim of this method is to angle and activate the bristles so that they penetrate and clean subgingivally. Research has shown that in relatively healthy individuals the bristles may penetrate up to 3 mm into the gingival crevice, although in a patient with inflammatory periodontal disease and reduced gingival tone, deeper penetration may occur (Figure 7.3b).

The bristles of the brush are pointed in an apical direction and then placed on the dentogingival junction at an angle of 45° to the long axis of the tooth. The brush is then activated by vibration in an anteroposterior direction or by small circular movements. The former method is the easier to perform, especially in the posterior quadrants. To clean the lingual surfaces of the anterior teeth requires the brush to be used in a vertical position, particularly in those patients with a very narrow dental arch.

Patients with marked gingival inflammation should be advised to brush very gently for the first few days after adopting this method so that the swollen tissues are not too severely abraded. They should avoid a hard brush.

Advantages
Disrupts plaque at and under the gingival margin. This method has good penetration of embrasure area and does not require a high degree of manual dexterity.

Disadvantages
Excessive pressure will cause gingival abrasion and soreness which may be limited by the use of a soft brush. It is also a time consuming technique.

The Roll method
In this method the bristles are moved with a sweeping action down from the gingiva onto the tooth (Figure 7.4).

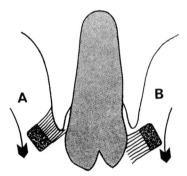

Figure 7.4   The Roll method of brushing. The bristles are pointed up towards the apex of the tooth on the overlying gingiva and pressure applied. They are then swept downwards over the gingiva and tooth. Subgingival cleaning is unlikely to occur

The head of the brush is placed against the surface of the tooth with the bristles pointing apically beyond the mucogingival junction. Pressure is applied against the gingiva and the handle of the brush rotated so that the bristles are swept over the dentogingival area onto the tooth. This basic action may be followed by a variety of other movements such as vibratory.

This method is relatively complicated and requires a degree of manual dexterity. There is some evidence that it is one of the least efficient brushing methods but modifications of this method may be useful in patients with areas of gingival recession.

Advantages
Considerable pressure may be applied to the tooth without the risk of causing gingival recession or abrasion. Gives stimulation to the gingiva, if one considers this to be of any importance.

Disadvantages
Requires considerable manual dexterity and a degree of wrist flexibility. Because of this it is not suitable for those with manual limitation, such as arthritics. It does not clean subgingivally or even at the gingival margin where there is any degree of gingival swelling, and is considered the least efficient of current brushing techniques.

Dentifrices

A dentifrice or toothpaste can be used in combination with brushing for the purpose of facilitating plaque removal and also as a method of applying therapeutic agents to the tooth surface for preventive or desensitizing purposes. The abrasive material in a dentifrice should have a particle hardness which does not produce wear of the tooth surface but facilitates stain and plaque removal. It has been shown that stained pellicle develops in subjects using a non-abrasive dentifrice.

For denture plaque removal a specifically made denture dentifrice should be recommended, using as the abrasive methylmethacrylate beads which will not abrade standard denture acrylic as would occur with standard dentifrices.

Desensitizing dentifrices tend to have a very low abrasive index and this is important as their main function is to produce a lowering of the sensitivity of exposed root dentine. When used continuously they may allow the development of stained pellicle, so their use should be interspersed with a standard toothpaste. The therapeutic agents used in commercial toothpastes to produce desensitization include strontium chloride, potassium chloride, potassium acetate, formaldehyde and various fluorides. The preventive compounds incorporated in dentifrices are fluoride compounds in the main, although chlorhexidine is now available in this form and more recently the 'tartar control' materials containing sodium pyrophosphate have become available. These calculus-reducing dentifrices would appear to be indicated for patients who form calculus very rapidly.

Ingredients of dentifrices
Each of the ingredients in toothpastes has a specific function and the major one is a polishing agent which may constitute up to 40% of the volume. The commonest polishing agents used are: calcium carbonate, calcium pyro-

phosphate, sodium metaphosphate, silica, zirconium silicate and dicalcium phosphate.

The dentifrice will also contain up to 30% humectant, which absorbs water and keeps the material moist by preventing it hardening on exposure to air. The commoner ones used are glycerol, sorbitol and propylene glycol. Flavouring agents are used to provide the taste and may be added in a level of up to 5%. Peppermint and spearmint flavourings are commonly used but a large variety of others in various combinations are often present. Up to 5% of the dentifrice may be stabilizing agents used to hold the material together and prevent it from separating into solid and liquid phases. As in icecream, alginates are used to fulfil this function. To lower the surface tension of the plaque and so assist in its removal, detergents are added and these give the typical foaming action. Preservatives are used to prevent the growth of micro-organisms and benzoates are a popular choice.

Fluoride is now added to the majority of dentifrices for its anticaries effect and sodium fluoride and sodium monofluorophosphate in concentrations of up to 1% are commonly present. Chlorhexidine is used in some dentifrices in a similar concentration.

It should be obvious that with such a cocktail of chemicals present every effort should be made to prevent the ingestion of toothpaste, especially in the young. This precaution is easier to achieve when very small amounts of paste are added to the brush. Despite concern about young individuals ingesting too much of the fluoride ion, experiments have shown that little is retained and the majority passes harmlessly out of the gut.

Interdental cleansing

Brushing alone will not remove plaque in the interdental areas so further aids such as dental floss or tape, woodsticks, interproximal brushes or single tufted interspace brushes may be advised for those patients who are suffering from plaque-induced gingival inflammation (Figure 7.5). The choice of aid will depend upon the size and accessibility of the interproximal area and also on the ability of the patient to clean it.

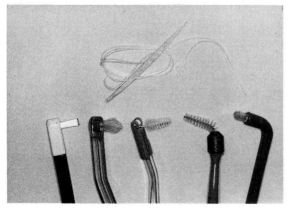

Figure 7.5   A range of items that may be used for interdental cleansing: above, dental tape and stick. Below from left to right: interspace and interdental brushes

The question is often asked at which age interdental cleaning should start. Young children would not possess the dexterity or motivation to undertake interdental cleansing, but this type of cleaning should begin once the permanent dentition has fully erupted in the teenage years. Dental floss or tape usage at this time could be very beneficial, particularly if there is a family history of susceptibility to inflammatory disease, although it is true to say that cooperation may be very variable at this age.

Floss and tape

In cases where the interdental papilla completely fills the embrasure space, effective plaque removal from interproximal tooth surfaces may be accomplished by the use of floss or tape. It has been shown that floss or tape may be placed subgingivally 2–3.5 mm below the tip of the papilla (Figure 7.6).

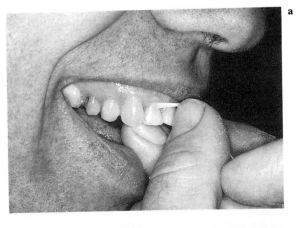

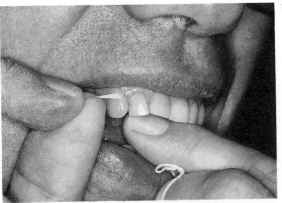

Figure 7.6 Dental tape in use: (a) the tape has been taken through the contact point and wrapped around the distal of the lateral incisor and moved subgingivally to clean this surface; (b) the tape has now been moved over the contact point, wrapped around the mesial of the canine to clean this surface

There are two main methods of use. In the commonest method about 40 cm are taken and wound around the two middle fingers with the bulk placed on one of these fingers (Figure 7.7a). As the floss or tape is used and soiled it is unwound from one finger to the other. In the second method the floss is tied in a loop (Figure 7.8a) which is then wound around the fingers as shown (Figure 7.8b). This method makes the material less likely to slip during use. Figure 7.7a, b and c shows the manipulation required when using floss or tape.

The technique of using floss is illustrated in Figure 7.6a and b, and involves its careful manipulation through the contact point and then moving the taut floss in an apico-occlusal direction over the whole of the mesial tooth surface to render it plaque-free. The floss is then moved over the interdental papilla to the adjacent distal tooth surface and the procedure repeated. A new section of floss should be used for each interdental space to minimize the chances of transferring micro-organisms from one site to another in the

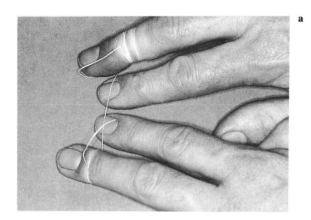

a

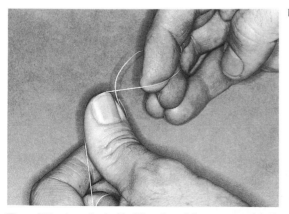

b

Figure 7.7   A method of holding dental floss or tape: (a) 40 cm are taken and wound around the two middle fingers with the bulk on one, to allow this to be unwound when the working area becomes soiled or frayed; (b) and (c) the thumbs and index fingers are used to control the floss or tape (see page 84)

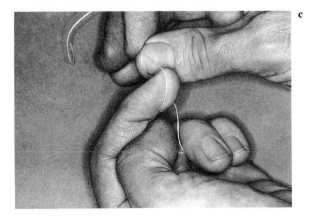

Figure 7.7 (*continued*)

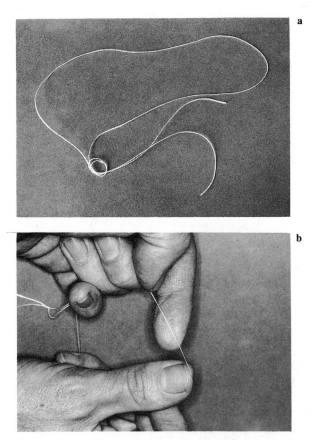

Figure 7.8   The loop method of using floss or tape: (a) about 20 cm are tied in a loop, as shown; (b) the loop is passed around the fingers of both hands and the thumb and an index finger used for control

mouth. There would appear to be little differences between the cleaning abilities of waxed or unwaxed floss, but patients with crowded teeth or interproximal restorations may prefer waxed types as it is easier to manipulate and has a reduced tendency to fray.

A variety of floss holders are available to make its use easier for patients with limited manual dexterity (Figure 7.9).

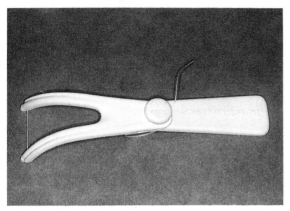

Figure 7.9   A floss or tape holder that can be used by a patient with limited manual dexterity

Superfloss, which is specially thickened in its middle area, may be indicated for larger interdental spaces where papillary recession has occurred or tissue loss is evident, such as around bridgework or following periodontal surgery (Figure 7.10). It can also be used to apply desensitizing dentifrices to exposed interdental root surfaces.

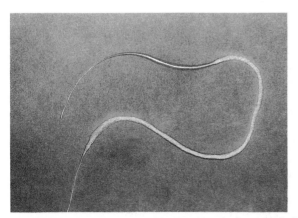

Figure 7.10   Superfloss, a modified flossing device suitable for cleaning large interdental spaces, crown or bridgework and implant abutments

Interdental points

These may be made of soft wood or plastic and in general take less time than floss to use and also require less manual dexterity. They are triangular in cross-section to fit into the interproximal space and are used with a pull/push action across the space, with the flat base positioned gingivally and the tip pointing occlusally. If they are to be recommended then their use is probably restricted to the older patient with some papillary recession.

Interproximal brushes

These brushes are indicated where there are wide interproximal spaces such as those seen after periodontal surgery or where recession has occurred. They are manufactured in a variety of sizes and shapes and some are supplied with handles (Figures 7.11 and 7.12). They may be very useful for cleaning around precision attachments and osseointegrated implant abutments. As a general rule they are used in the same situations as interdental

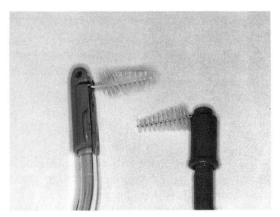

Figure 7.11 Interproximal brushes, useful for interdental cleaning where there are open embrasure spaces. May also be called interdental brushes

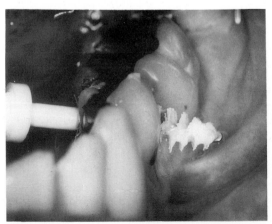

Figure 7.12 An interproximal brush used to clean between two large restorations which have been contoured to permit easy access of the brush

points but are more efficient as the bristles allow greater contact with the tooth surfaces, especially when difficult contours such as concavities are present.

Single tuft brushes
These are often called interspace brushes and are designed to clean in difficult areas such as between crowded teeth or around bridgework. They are also useful in reaching the buccal and lingual surfaces of posterior teeth that prove difficult to clean with a standard toothbrush (Figure 7.13).

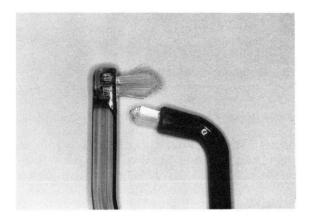

Figure 7.13   A single tuft or interspace brush. Useful for cleaning irregular spaces

Chemical control of plaque

Considerable interest over the past two decades has been directed to this area, with various antiseptics being investigated and more recently a number of drugs. The degree of success with regard to supragingival plaque control has been variable. The antiplaque agent has been delivered by a variety of methods such as mouthwashes, toothpastes and chewing gum. Antiseptics, enzyme preparations and surface energy reducing agents have all been tried. Combating the subgingival microflora has proved more difficult and the methods tried have included placing antiseptics, such as chlorhexidine, or antibiotics such as tetracycline, into periodontal pockets by means of a local sustained delivery device such as acrylic or cellulose gels. The incorporated active agent is released over a period of days after contact with moisture.

Antiseptics

The antiseptics that have been shown to possess antiplaque properties include cetylpyridinium chloride, sanguinarine, benzalkonium chloride and various zinc salts, but the chemical that has been most successful is chlorhexidine in its gluconate or acetate form. The use of chlorhexidine has been shown to be effective at plaque prevention in numerous studies since the initial work by Loe and Random-Schiott in 1970 using groups of dental students. Chlorhexidine is considered to be particularly effective because it is adsorbed onto the surfaces of teeth, pellicle and the oral mucosa and is released slowly over a long period of time, thereby having a prolonged disruptive effect on the micro-organisms that make up plaque.

Antiseptics are very useful adjuncts in the control of dental plaque. Initially research in the use of chlorhexidine concentrated on its value in the reduction of plaque and periodontal inflammation, but more recently attention has been directed to its use in the control of dental caries. It has been shown in a group of caries-prone children that it was possible to slow the incidence of carious attack by the regular use of chlorhexidine gel in a custom-made vinyl applicator worn for 5 minutes daily, over a period of 14 days and repeated every 4 months, if the salivary *Streptococcus mutans* counts rose above a predetermined threshold.

Combinations of chlorhexidine and fluoride have been found to be very useful in controlling plaque levels and caries susceptibility in patients who have received radiotherapy to tumours near the salivary glands. Another method of delivering chlorhexidine and other chemicals is by means of an oral irrigator. This device delivers a pulsed jet of fluid which can be directed into areas of the mouth that are difficult to clean and is also useful for patients with intermaxillary fixation for immobilization of fractured jaws. Another technique that some recommend is irrigation of periodontal pockets with chlorhexidine in a syringe with a blunt needle.

Despite its undoubted usefulness, chlorhexidine has a number of disadvantages, the main ones of which are as follows:

1. *Staining*. This is caused by chlorhexidine denaturing the protein pellicle deposited on the teeth. This denatured pellicle is more susceptible to food stains such as are present in tea and coffee. By avoiding these and limiting the use of chlorhexidine to 4 weeks followed by professional cleaning, the problem may be controlled.
2. *Taste*. The natural taste of chlorhexidine is very bitter and flavouring agents are used to mask its immediate impact. Despite this there may be interference with taste perception for up to 24 hours.
3. *Mucosal irritation*. This has been reported in a small number of patients and is thought to be due to the mucosal surface adsorption of chlorhexidine.
4. *Parotid swelling*. A few cases of parotid swelling have been reported which resolved on stopping use of the mouthrinse.

Removal of deposits

The acquired deposits that are found adhering to tooth surfaces are salivary pellicle, dental plaque, calculus and a variety of stains. Scaling is the procedure by which these deposits are removed from the tooth surface. Although the significance of salivary pellicle and its relationship to dental disease is unclear – it probably has a protective function – both dental plaque and calculus are associated with inflammatory periodontal disease. Scaling differs from root planing in that the latter procedure consists of instrumentation not only to remove surface deposits, but also to smooth the root surface and remove a thin layer of cementum, thus reducing the endotoxin burden. Some authorities do not feel that effective scaling can be carried out subgingivally unless followed by root planing.

It is probable that root planing reduces the level of cementum-bound endotoxin to a biologically acceptable level and thus allows healing of the adjacent periodontal soft tissues. However, recent work has shown that endotoxin may be reduced to the level seen on healthy root surfaces by very light root planing or even by polishing the root with a mild abrasive, providing that the root surface in the pocket is instrumented in a thorough, systematic way. It may well be that the only differences between scaling and root planing is the overall reduction in root surface contaminants, and this has to be less in some patients than in others who have decreased resistance to the influence of dental plaque and its by-products. There are, of course, differences in the instruments used in scaling (which is often a supragingival procedure) and root planing (which is always carried out in subgingival sites).

Principles of control of tooth deposits

The three fundamentals which allow effective control of acquired tooth surface deposits are their detection, adequate removal and the prevention of recurrence.

Calculus deposits may be detected by visual and tactile methods. Visual detection can be aided by a stream of air directed at the gingival margin from the triple syringe, thus drying out supragingival calculus which will lighten and appear chalky against the tooth surface. Subgingival calculus may appear as a dark ring often visible through the overlying gingiva and deflecting the gingival margin with the air syringe will reveal these deposits directly (Figure 7.14).

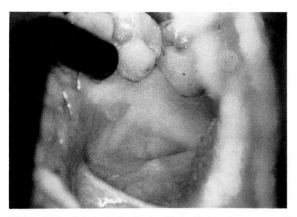

Figure 7.14 Subgingival calculus lingually to a lower premolar which has been revealed by directing a stream of air against the tooth

A variety of probes may be used to feel for calculus within the periodontal pocket and the two most useful are the World Health Organization 622 probe and the Cross calculus probe (Figure 7.15). Both these probes are able to detect the roughness of calculus when they are run over the root surface and they will usually catch beneath the apical edge of the deposits.

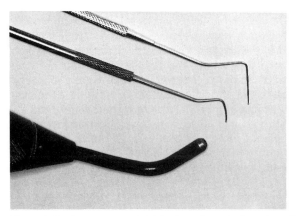

Figure 7.15 Instruments useful in detecting calculus: the WHO probe, the Cross calculus probe and the triple syringe

Parts of an instrument

All hand instruments consist of three basic sections: the handle, the shank and the working tip (Figure 7.16).

Modern scaling and root planing instruments have balanced grip handles, which give better distribution of weight and a large area of contact for the fingers. Often the handle is hollow which, besides reducing the weight, is claimed to give greater tactile discrimination.

The shank is that part of the instrument which connects the working tip to the handle. The angle and length of the shank determines the access obtained by the tip to the tooth surface.

The working tip contains the cutting edge or edges which remove the acquired deposits. Scalers are classified according to the shape of the tip and there are five basic designs: (a) sickles, (b) hoes, (c) files, (d) push (or chisel), and (e) curettes.

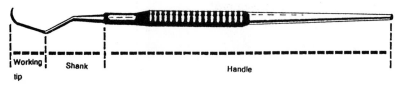

Figure 7.16 Parts of an instrument: working tip, shank and handle

Theoretical basis of scaling

During scaling a sharp working edge is placed on the tooth surface adjacent to the calculus and moved along that surface to dislodge the calculus. The angle at which the working tip is held against the tooth surface is important as scaling is more efficient if the tip leans back from the direction of movement than if it leans forward; however, in practice most scaling is performed with the tip at 90° or less to the tooth surface. This angle is called the rake angle and is positive if the instrument tip leans back and negative when it leans forward (Figure 7.17). In practice one cannot usually achieve more than 20° positive rake angle because the thickness of the scaling instrument will prevent further angulation. The angle between the non-working lateral surface of the scaler and the tooth is the clearance angle. It is necessary to have a clearance angle because without it there will be no 'bite' into the calculus.

Instrument grip
The instrument should be held in the correct way as this will determine the amount of control and thus the stability and effectiveness in use. There are three possible ways to hold a scaler:

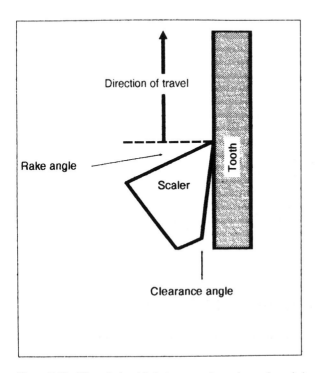

Figure 7.17   The relationship between scaler, rake angle and clearance angle

1. Standard pen grip (Figure 7.18).
2. Modified pen grip (Figure 7.19).
3. Palm grip (Figure 7.20).

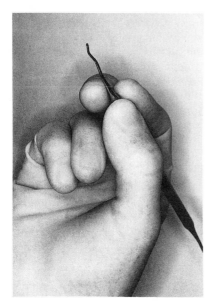

Figure 7.18   The standard pen grip

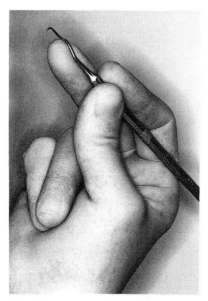

Figure 7.19   The modified pen grip, with middle finger used to support and stabilize the instrument

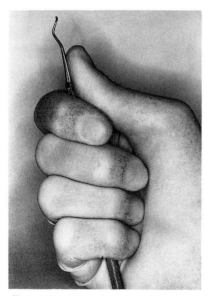

Figure 7.20   The palm grip, which gives increased force but poor control of the instrument

Standard pen grip
The instrument is held between the thumb and index finger and the medial part of the middle finger is used to control its movement. This grip is not commonly used.

Modified pen grasp
This modification of the standard pen grip is used for many procedures. Instead of the side of the medial surface of the middle finger being used, the terminal pad is utilized on the shank of the instrument, giving increased control.

Palm grip
On rare occasions during scaling the palm grip is used to give more power, but at the price of decreased control and visibility. The handle of the instrument is held in the palm of the hand with the fingers grasping the handle and the thumb placed on the shank to control movement.

As well as an appropriate instrument grip it is also important to establish a finger rest to ensure stability and lessen the possibility of slipping when applying pressure. The third or ring finger is the main source of the finger rest and the fourth or small finger are often used in addition (Figure 7.21). These fingers may rest as follows (in order of preference):

(a) on the tooth being scaled (Figure 7.21a);
(b) on the adjacent teeth (Figure 7.21b);
(c) on teeth in the same jaw, but some distance away (Figure 7.21c);
(d) on teeth in the opposite jaw (Figure 7.21d);

(e) on the external soft tissues overlying bone, for example on the patient's chin (Figure 7.21e);

(f) in difficult cases, the fingers of the non-working hand may be rested and the finger rest placed on these (Figure 7.21f).

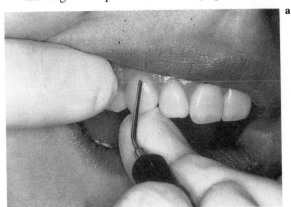

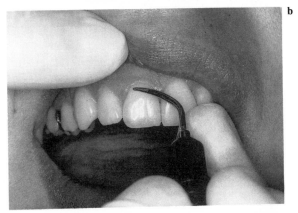

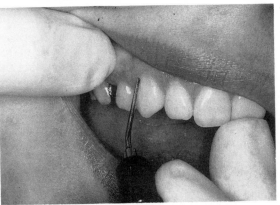

Figure 7.21 Finger rests that may be used when scaling in order of preference: (a) on tooth being scaled; (b) on adjacent tooth; (c) on remote tooth; (d) on teeth in the opposite jaw; (e) on the patient's chin; (f) on the fingers of the non-working hand

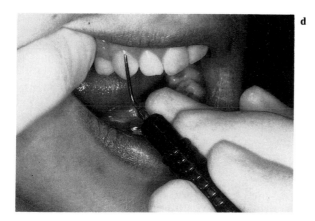

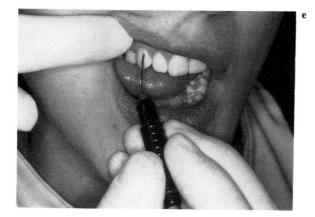

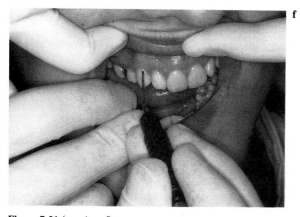

Figure 7.21 (*continued*)

Working position

Most dental procedures including scaling are undertaken with the patient in a near horizontal position, which gives the seated operator the ability to perform most of the work using direct vision. However, working with a horizontal patient does require three important precautions to be taken:

1. Eyesight protection must be provided.
2. The airway must be watched carefully and protection in the form of a butterfly sponge used if necessary.
3. Some method of moisture control will usually be required.

From a seated position it should be possible for a right-handed operator working in the 10 o'clock position behind the patient with the patient's feet in the six o'clock position, to instrument all the areas of the mouth under direct vision with the exception of the upper right palatal and the very posterior teeth on the right buccal segment. For these two areas it will often be necessary to move to the front of the patient and work facing the back of the unit.

Unfortunately, it is far from rare for dental professionals to develop back and limb problems, many caused by poor working practices. Although it must be admitted that some individuals are more susceptible to these postural problems, many could be avoided by adopting sensible working positions. The fundamental requirements for good working posture have been covered in other texts and reference to the publications by J. E. Paul is recommended. The main requirements for comfortable operating are:

1. Be seated comfortably without stress or bodily distortion.
2. Have as much of the working area in direct vision as possible.
3. Be able to reach the working area and the instrument delivery system without excessive movement or strain.

For these conditions to apply, attention must be given to both the posture of the operator and the position of the patient. Let us consider each separately.

Operator posture
It is generally agreed that all dental operations, with few exceptions, can and should be undertaken with the operator seated. There are, however, some patients such as the elderly, those in an advanced stage of pregnancy or those with various hernias, who require to be treated in an upright position and this may oblige the operator to work standing. The ideal position of the operator for seated dentistry is shown in Figure 7.22 and the following should be observed:

1. The back should be straight and self-supporting.
2. The height of the chair should allow the feet to be placed flat on the floor so that the upper thighs are sloping downwards at no more than 15°.
3. The back of the operating chair should allow the legs to part with a space of no more than 30 cm between the knees.
4. The operator's head should be tilted downward at the angle at which they would usually read a newspaper, often about 15°.

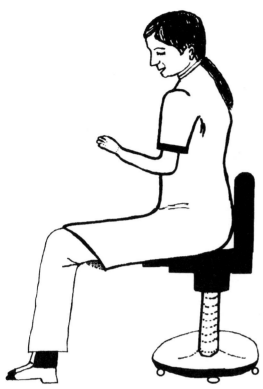

Figure 7.22 The ideal position for seated dentistry. The back is straight and upper thighs sloping slightly downwards. The head is tilted down about 15° and the working distance is about 30 cm

5. The patient's head should be at the distance of comfortable focus, usually about 30 cm from the eyes, which is approximately at the operator's midsternal level.

For the operator to work in this manner the position of the patient is also important, not only for the convenience of the operator but also for the comfort and safety of the patient. The preferred position is for the patient to be horizontal, as it has been shown that in this position the back of the tongue provides a seal against the soft palate, making the ingestion or inhalation of small objects or water less likely. The main characteristics of the patient position are as follows:

1. The patient should be fully horizontal with the body supported by the padded dental chair. It is particularly important that the shoulders are fully supported and that there is no space between the back element and the seat of the chair.
2. The headrest should be flat with a small concavity to support the head but allow rotation when required. This will permit maximum visibility for the operator.
3. The dental chair must be able to be rapidly adjusted in an emergency to place the patient in the Trendelenberg position, with the lower limbs above that of the trunk.

Instrumentation: general rules

The successful practice of periodontics depends not only upon the ability to motivate patients in the daily use of effective oral hygiene, but also in the skilful use of instruments during scaling and root planing. For many patients these procedures may be undertaken without any form of anaesthesia. In some cases, however, especially when carrying out root planing, some analgesia will be required. Often the use of a topical anaesthetic cream will suffice, particularly when at least 2 min are allowed to elapse between application and scaling, so that maximum anaesthesia is achieved. When topical anaesthesia is inadequate, block or infiltration anaesthesia will be required; some patients will need even this reinforcing with inhalation relative analgesia.

The following ten rules will help to improve the efficiency of instrumentation:

1. Be comfortable. Ensure that both you and the patient are seated comfortably.
2. Position yourself for maximum visibility. If possible work with the site in direct vision with a good, well-adjusted operating light.
3. Follow an orderly sequence of instrument use and make sure they are laid out in the order of use *before* and *after* application. This will help to avoid the time wasted in searching for instruments on an untidy worktop.
4. Use as few instruments as possible and know the function of each instrument.
5. Maintain control of instruments during use not only to prevent inefficient scaling but also traumatic damage caused by slipping – good finger rests are essential.
6. Maintain a clear field by use of cotton wool rolls and aspiration. Both haemorrhage and saliva will require control.
7. Ensure your instruments are sharp and serviceable.
8. Use a slow, deliberate and methodical approach but do not confuse roughness with thoroughness.
9. Always talk to the patient in a friendly and sympathetic manner, not only on completion of the task but during the procedure. This ensures that the patient adjusts to the procedure even if they found it difficult and time consuming.
10. Always clean up the patient before they leave the surgery. This is a courtesy appreciated by all patients.

Hand instruments

The sickle scaler
This is a generic term which includes all scalers with a working tip projecting from the shank at approximately a right angle and having a sharp pointed end (Figures 7.23 and 7.24). The method of use may be by pulling, such as

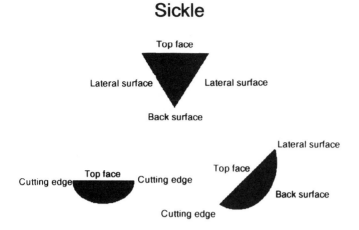

Figure 7.23 A comparison of the working tips of a sickle, universal and site specific curette

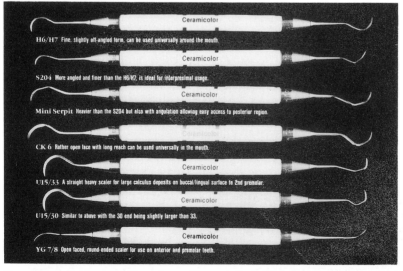

Figure 7.24 A range of sickle scalers, with use indicated (courtesy of Ash Instrument Division, Dentsply Plc)

the Jaquette No. 1 or rotation of the handle (Jaquettes 2 and 3 and Hygienist sickles). They have two cutting edges which are formed by the convergence of the top surface and the two lateral surfaces. The cross-section of the working tip is triangular in shape.

Uses
Mainly for supragingival scaling. A sickle may also be used to scale or root plane just beneath to the gingival margin, provided the gingival pocket is fairly loose. This instrument should not be inserted too deeply into a pocket as the sharp tip will lacerate the soft tissue wall.

Method of use
The cutting edge is placed against the tooth if possible with a positive rake angle, but 90° is an acceptable compromise. It is then moved up the tooth with a pull stroke.

The periodontal hoe
This has a straight cutting edge on a short wide blade projecting at right angles from the shaft.

Uses
The hoe is the principal instrument for removing heavy deposits of sub-gingival calculus from beneath the gingiva and for root planing. It may also be used to remove heavy deposits of supragingival calculus. Hoes such as those in the MacFarlane set are suitable for scaling mesially, distally, facially and lingually whilst modified hoes (Figures 7.25 and 7.26) are useful for scaling and root planing in furcations.

Method of use
The working tip is slid down the root surface over the calculus until the bottom edge is palpated. Pressure is applied to hold the hoe against the deposits and the shank against the crown. The instrument is then moved towards the crown to plane away the calculus.

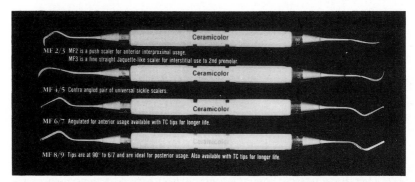

Figure 7.25   MacFarlane scaling and root planing set. The hoes included in this set are suitable for scaling and root planing on facial, lingual, mesial and distal aspects of teeth (courtesy of Ash Instrument Division, Dentsply Plc)

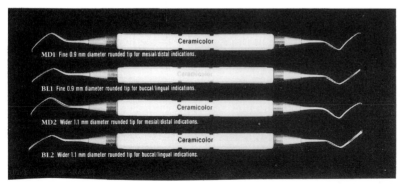

Figure 7.26   A set of modified periodontal hoes suitable for scaling in furcations (courtesy of Ash Instrument Division, Dentsply Plc)

The periodontal file

The file has a series of cutting edges set at right angles to the shank on a round, oval or rectangular base (Figures 7.27 and 7.28).

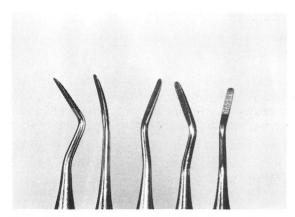

Figure 7.27   A set of Bunting files suitable for root planing in loose pockets after the removal of gross calculus deposits

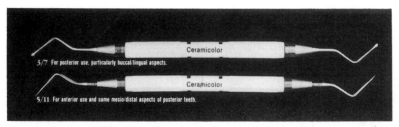

Figure 7.28   A set of Hirschfeld files suitable for root planing in tight pockets (courtesy of Ash Instrument Division, Dentsply Plc)

Uses

The file is used for subgingival scaling and root planing, but will not cope with heavy deposits which must be removed with a hoe scaler first.

Method of use

The instrument is slid down the root surface to the lower edge of the calculus. Pressure is applied to hold the cutting edges and the shank against the tooth and the instrument moved towards the crown removing the deposits. The design of a file requires repeated strokes to be made whilst instrumenting an area.

The push scaler

The push or chisel scaler has a single straight bevelled cutting edge set at right angles to the shank (Figure 7.29).

Uses

The push scaler is used to remove heavy deposits of supragingival calculus from the interdental surfaces of the anterior teeth. It should only be used when the embrasure spaces are open and sufficient space is present.

Method of use

The cutting edge is placed from the labial aspect against the tooth surface and pressure applied to cleave away adhering calculus deposits.

The dental curette

This has a spoon-shaped working tip with a curved cutting edge. There are two principal types, the universal with two cutting edges (Figure 7.30) and the site specific which has a cutting edge on one side only (Figures 7.31 and 7.32). A comparison of universal with site specific curettes is shown in Table 7.1.

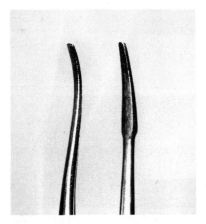

Figure 7.29   Push or chisel scalers

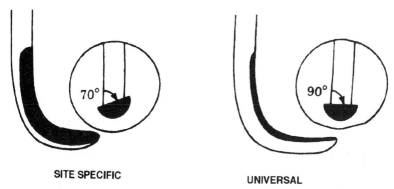

SITE SPECIFIC   **UNIVERSAL**

Figure 7.30 A comparison of a site specific curette, such as a Gracey, with a universal. The angle of the working tip to the shank is shown on the inset

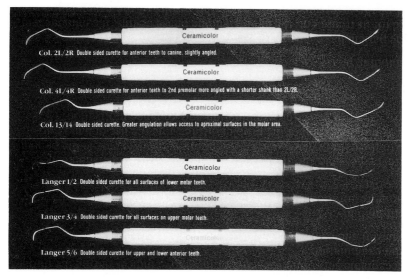

Figure 7.31 Universal curettes: Columbia and Langer (courtesy of Ash Instrument Division, Dentsply Plc)

Uses

The curette is the principal instrument for fine subgingival scaling, root planing and root surface smoothing. It may also be used for curetting the soft tissue wall of the pocket, a procedure called subgingival curettage.

Method of use

The working tip is inserted to the base of the pocket and tilted to give a positive rake angle. It is used with a pull stroke towards the occlusal surface.

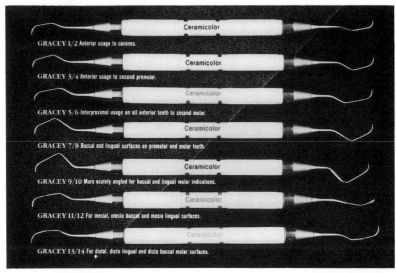

Figure 7.32   Gracey site specific curettes (courtesy of Ash Instrument Division, Dentsply Plc)

Table 7.1   Comparison of a universal curette with site specific

	Universal	*Site specific*
Use location	Universal: designed for all areas	Site specific: designed for different areas
Blade angle	Face of blade 90° to shank	Offset blade: face of blade 60° to shank
Edge curvature	Curved in one plane: blade curves up but not laterally	Curved in two planes: blade curves up and laterally
Use of working edges	Both edges used for instrumentation	Only one edge used for instrumentation
Advantages	Fewer instruments needed for scaling	More precise instrumentation of specific area

Mechanical scalers

Mechanical scalers are used in dentistry to remove plaque, calculus and stains from the teeth. The use of these automated scaling instruments makes the work of the operator so much easier and for many patients makes the scaling procedure more acceptable. Although it is said that these scalers cannot perform root planing, they have a valuable role in the removal of gross deposits and flushing out the pocket. Ultrasonic scalers operate above 20 kHz and sonic scalers in the 5–10 kHz range. Both types of instrument need a water spray as heat is produced during use at the working tip and the cooling spray has the additional advantage of washing away dislodged deposits, but also the distinct disadvantage of producing an aerosol (Figure 7.33). Table 7.2 lists some of the types of mechanical scaler classified according to the method used to produce tip vibration, and identifies the manufacturer.

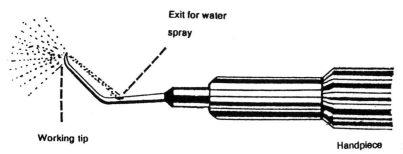

Figure 7.33   The working area of a mechanical scaler showing the relationship of water exit to working tip

Table 7.2   Mechanical scalers classified according to the technique used to produce vibration. The manufacturer is also indicated

Ultrasonic	
Magnetostrictive	
Cavitron:	Dentsply International, York, USA
Odontosonic:	A/S L Goof, Horsholm, Denmark
Scaletron:	Dental Supply Co Ltd, London, UK
Piezo-electronic	
Piezon:	EMS PA, Le Sentier, Switzerland
Sonic	
Enac:	Osada Electric Co Ltd, Tokyo, Japan
Kavo Soniflex:	Kavo Dental Ltd, Amersham, UK
Micro-Mega:	Prodonta SA, Geneva, Switzerland
Titan:	Star Dental Products, Valley Forge, USA

Types of mechanical scalers

Ultrasonic instruments
These operate at above the frequency of human hearing, usually between 20 000 and 30 000 vibrations per second (20–30 kHz). There are two different types available on the market:

1. Magnetostrictive types. These use a core or stack of ferromagnetic material which is acted upon by electrical windings in the handpiece which produce an alternating magnetic flux. When the stack is magnetized it contracts and as the stack is connected to the working tip this mechanical change is relayed to the tooth surface.
2. Piezoelectronic types. These utilize the ability of small currents to alter the dimensions of a quartz crystal to produce the vibration.

Air or sonic scalers
Sonic scalers are operated by the air line usually connected to the air turbine. This is passed over a reed in the handpiece which then vibrates in a similar manner to a musical instrument. Sonic scalers operate at frequencies below that of the limit of hearing, typically in the 5–7 kHz range.

A comparison of the characteristics of ultrasonic and sonic scalers is shown in Table 7.3.

Table 7.3   Comparison of ultrasonic and sonic scalers

Ultrasonic	Sonic
Electrically powered	Air powered
Oscillatory pattern governed by tip design	Oscillatory pattern usually circular
Not easily damped by loading	Easily damped by loading
Cavitation always present	Cavitation not always present
Acoustic streaming occurs	Acoustic streaming occurs
Expensive to purchase	Relatively cheap to purchase
Difficult to sterilize	Easy to sterilize
Contraindicated in patients with cardiac pacemakers	No contraindications

Method of action
The removal of calculus and other deposits is achieved in three ways:

1. *Mechanical abrading action.* The action is a mixture of back and forth and circulatory movements and this mechanically abrades and chips away at the deposits on the root surface. A variety of differing shaped tips is available to achieve this result. There are differences in the oscillatory patterns of ultrasonic and sonic scalers. The ultrasonic has a higher energy output and is not easily damped by loading. The sonic scaler has a larger and more coarse pattern of movement to compensate for the lower energy level and is more easily damped by high loading, although this may not be obvious to the operator. It is, however, easier to sterilize than the ultrasonic instrument.
2. *Cavitational effects.* These are usually seen with the ultrasonic scalers as the sonic variety do not as a general rule have sufficient energy output at the tip to cause cavitation. All mechanical scalers are provided with a flow of cooling water directed at the tip to remove any heat caused by

friction between the tip and the tooth surface. The water contains minute air bubbles which are expanded by the energy in the vibrating tip which causes them to have a negative internal pressure for a fraction of a second and then implode, releasing large shock waves. Such forces have been shown to remove plaque and calculus from the tooth surface.

One of the side effects of the water flow and cavitation is the generation of a large aerosol against which precautions should be taken, as described later.

3. *Acoustic streaming.* All mechanical scalers set up vigorous movements of the water around their tips and this is termed acoustic streaming. This assists in the removal of some of the tooth surface deposits and in the disruption of plaque colonies.

Principles of use

Modern mechanical scalers are self-tuning, although one may still find the older types of ultrasonic scaler which require to be tuned to give the maximum power output for any particular setting. The higher the power setting the greater the vibration and the more likely it is for the patient to experience discomfort. In general a medium setting should be used and this has the added advantage of reducing this risk of unwanted tooth surface damage.

The instrument should be positioned with the oscillating working tip almost in the long axis of the tooth with a very small rake angle. Light pressure should be applied and the tip kept constantly on the move with a light circulatory stroking action. The tip should not be held stationary in any one area for too long as this will cause excessive abrasion of the tooth in that area. Instrumentation should not be rushed and the surface should be checked from time to time for smoothness. This can be done with the tip without the power on.

Instrument tip selection

The use of an appropriate scaling tip is important if the task is to be carried out effectively. As in hand scaling, the heaviest tip design is used to remove the heaviest deposits. The type of calculus deposit that literally splints the teeth together may be removed with the chisel tip which dislodges the interdental calculus in a labiolingual direction, particularly on the anterior teeth. The gross supragingival deposit is then removed using the beaver-tail tip in all areas of the mouth but, because of its size and shape, it is not suitable for fine or deep deposits.

Once gross calculus has been removed then the universal tip may be used to remove fine deposits. This tip has no cutting edges and readily adapts to curved tooth surfaces but, because of its bulk, will not scale easily any lesion deeper than about 4 mm. For these areas a fine tip similar to a periodontal probe or heavy gauge needle is used (Figure 7.34). This will remove fine deposits and smooth the root surface and is particularly useful in furcations, root grooves and in concave areas such as the canine fossa of the maxillary first premolar.

The working movement of each tip is as follows:

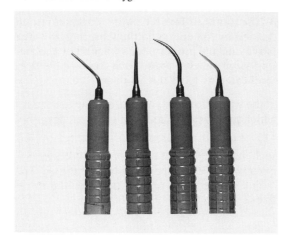

Figure 7.34   Useful tips for the ultrasonic scaler: from left to right, probe, chisel, universal and beaver-tail

Chisel: used in a labiolingual direction only;
Beaver-tail: horizontal strokes on the proximal surfaces and vertical strokes on labial and lingual surfaces;
Universal: vertical strokes interproximally and horizontal strokes buccally and lingually;
Probe tip: diagonal strokes from the lingual or labial aspect using a rapid short movement with each contact preferably less than 3 seconds.

Potential hazards of mechanical scalers
The most serious hazard from the operator's point of view is the considerable aerosol generated, especially by the ultrasonic machines. The operator should wear a good quality mask and protective spectacles, in addition to the usual gloves. The patient should be asked to rinse with an oral antiseptic such as chlorhexidine digluconate 0.2% for 1 minute before the procedure to reduce the oral flora, and a high volume aspirator used to remove the remaining aerosol. In view of these problems, an ultrasonic or sonic scaler should not be used with highly infectious patients such as those infected with human immunodeficiency or hepatitis B viruses.

The instrument produces a lot of unwanted noise and there is some evidence that an operator may suffer permanent hearing loss in the higher frequency range if it is used for long periods of time. The patient does not appear to suffer any permanent damage from this noise.

The tooth surface can be damaged by frictional heating if insufficient coolant is used and by abrasive scratching if the tip is incorrectly applied. Porcelain jacket crowns may be fractured by the tips and it is possible for a cement lute to be broken, so it is important to avoid contact of crown and bridgework with mechanical scalers.

A potential danger exists for patients fitted with an electronic cardiac pacemaker. The ultrasonic scaler is known to emit a large electromagnetic field which may interfere with the older types of pacemaker, and it is wise to avoid its use with this category of patient. More modern pacemakers are shielded and compensated to reduce this risk but it would be unwise to test the effectiveness of this in the dental chair. The field of interference is small, of the order of 1 metre, and is only likely to cause an effect on the patient being treated. Sonic scalers do not operate electrically so they have no effect on a pacemaker.

Comparison of mechanical and hand instruments

The mechanical scaler is said to be quicker and easier for the operator, and has been shown to reduce hand fatigue and strain. The water flow flushes out pockets and removes debris during scaling. Visibility may be improved by the washed field effect. It has been concluded by several researchers that the use of a mechanical scaler can produce a similar root finish to that achieved by a hand instrument but this will obviously vary with the skill of the operator. In clinical use ultrasonic or sonic scaling is, in any case, always followed by hand scaling.

A greater potential for damage exists, especially if the equipment is misused. Some patients will find mechanical scalers uncomfortable in use, especially if exposed cervical dentine is present. The lack of tactile sensation may also be a problem, particularly if visibility is hampered by the water spray. The equipment is expensive and like all mechanical items prone to breakdown. Despite these drawbacks it is generally agreed that their use is to be routinely recommended for most scaling and root planing procedures.

Recent ultrasonic innovations

Recent changes in ultrasonic instruments include some operating at the higher frequency of 30 kHz instead of the previously common 25 kHz and the ability to pass a chemical solution through the tip to permit therapeutic irrigation during scaling, as used in the Dentsply Cavi-Med system (Figure 7.35). Although the system has not yet been fully evaluated, early research results show considerable promise.

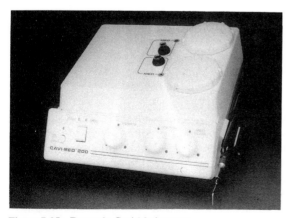

Figure 7.35 Dentsply Cavi-Med system

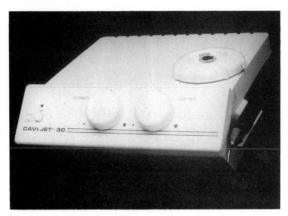

Figure 7.36   Dentsply Cavi-Jet system

Another recently developed system is the Cavi-Jet (Figure 7.36). After scaling, a jet of air containing an abrasive material is passed through the tip to remove any remaining plaque and stain.

Supragingival scaling

The removal of supragingival deposits of dental calculus is most efficiently achieved with an ultrasonic or sonic scaler. This should be applied gently to the tooth surface and moved with small overlapping or circular strokes to remove the deposits. If a mechanical scaler is not available, or the patient cannot tolerate it, or if the patient has a medical condition such as HIV infection which contraindicates the use of a mechanical scaler, the following hand instruments may be employed.

A large excavator or Cumine scaler will remove large accumulations of calculus. The push scaler can then be used between the lower incisor teeth to remove interdental deposits. A Sickle or Jaquette scaler can be used on the lingual and interdental areas, and finally an appropriate hoe will remove facial and lingual calculus.

The removal of supragingival calculus is often combined with subgingival scaling.

Subgingival scaling

Supragingival scaling ideally should be completed before subgingival scaling, as the presence of deposits on the crown of the tooth will hinder visibility and prevent the correct application of the scaler to the root.

Before activating the instrument a series of exploratory strokes should be made to determine the location and topography of subgingival deposits. A scaling instrument or WHO probe is passed down the root surface to the base of the pocket. If any apparent obstruction is felt, the instrument is moved out from the root surface and gently extended apically to distinguish between a ledge of calculus or the junctional epithelium. As a general rule, calculus will feel hard and the junctional epithelium soft and springy.

When the pocket and deposits have been mentally mapped out, scaling can commence. The best instrument to start with is the ultrasonic scaler. This will dislodge and flush out the larger deposits. Following this a hoe scaler is used to continue the scaling, working round the site in a methodical, overlapping manner. Finally dental curettes are used to remove fine deposits and leave a smooth root surface.

Following the scaling the pocket should be flushed with the triple syringe or the spray from an ultrasonic scaler to remove any retained particles or micro-organisms.

Root planing

Root planing is indicated when, in the presence of good supragingival plaque control and following the removal of all clinically detectable sub-gingival deposits, the activity of a periodontal pocket persists. The aims of root planing are to:

(a) Remove a thin layer of endotoxin-laden cementum;
(b) remove all deposits of plaque and calculus; and
(c) leave the root surface clinically smooth.

If these aims are achieved then the root surface should be rendered biologically inert and the persistent periodontal lesion begin to resolve.

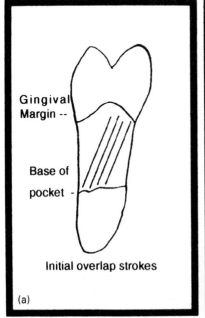 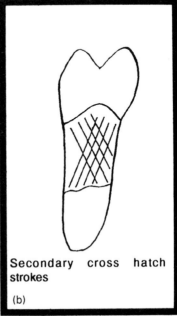

Figure 7.37 Technique for root planing: (a) initial overlapping strokes; (b) secondary cross hatch strokes. This method allows each area to be covered on four occasions by the instrument.

For the majority of patients local anaesthesia will be required for the teeth to be root planed. In the maxilla this will require the use of infiltration techniques but in the mandible block anaesthesia is necessary.

Instrumentation during root planing is very similar to that used during subgingival scaling, but the technique is more exacting, although often there is no calculus to remove. It is again worthwhile to commence and finish with an ultrasonic scaler as there is some evidence of improved healing following its use. The hand instruments are then used in the following order:

1. Hoe scalers to remove calculus and some cementum.
2. Periodontal files to continue the root surface removal.
3. Curettes to remove fine deposits, reach into inaccessible areas such as furcations, and leave a smooth root surface.

The method of use of instruments also varies from scaling. The initial strokes should be made from the base of the pocket up the root surface with an overlapping technique as shown in Figure 7.37. This should be followed by a consolidating series of movements at 45° to the initial strokes. In this manner the root surface is quartered by the instrument and the majority of the contaminated cementum removed. The pocket is then flushed with the water spray to remove loosened deposits. This may be achieved by using the ultrasonic scaler provided care is taken not to further roughen the root surface following the hand smoothing. Finally the pocket is irrigated with an antiplaque agent such as 0.2% chlorhexidine digluconate.

Contraindications to root planing are poor patient motivation, teeth of a hopeless prognosis, severe dentinal sensitivity (which will be worsened by the procedure) and the presence of acute infection.

Chapter 8

Chronic periodontal diseases

Recent epidemiological evidence indicates that between 10% and 20% of the world's population is highly susceptible to some form of destructive periodontal disease. A further 40% are likely to suffer from milder, but no less troublesome forms of plaque-induced periodontal diseases. Although these findings by and large apply to populations without access to effective health care, even if a smaller percentage of our population is at risk, they still present a considerable challenge to our ability to treat their disease and meet their expectations – expectations which will be considerably greater than those of undeveloped populations.

In any large dental practice many patients will present every day with some form of periodontal disease. This disease will vary from early forms of gingivitis, as is frequently seen in children and adolescents, to advanced periodontitis, the prevalence of which rises markedly in the fourth and fifth decades of life. Although there may be disagreement as to the most effective way to treat these periodontal diseases, there is universal agreement that the two most important elements are the control of tooth surface deposits and their removal, but the application of these principles will vary according to the presentation of the disease.

Management of gingivitis

Gingivitis is characterized by superficial inflammation of the gingival tissues with no loss of epithelial attachment, although swelling may cause false pocketing to be present. It is the one type of periodontal disease that has been categorically shown to be related to the oral hygiene of the patient. The severity of gingivitis may vary from a slight change in texture and colour of the gingival margin, to an intense erythema with a tendency to spontaneous bleeding following minor trauma. Although it is usually a chronic inflammatory process, acute exacerbations are common. This chapter will only deal with the management of chronic gingivitis, the acute forms being described later in the book.

Early gingivitis may be completely reversed by an improvement in the standard of dental home care, providing there are no factors present such as deficient restorations or calculus that make plaque removal difficult. Later stages may pose more complex problems such as gingival hyperplasia, which will sometimes need surgical removal. The key factor in the management of all types of periodontal disease is, again, effective home care of the mouth.

However, it is insufficient to merely instruct a patient on how to brush and clean interdentally. Indeed any suggestion that it is the patient's fault and that they have a 'dirty' mouth may not persuade them to clean more efficiently, but may have the opposite effect by arousing antagonism.

There are a number of obstacles that have to be successfully negotiated before one can achieve the restoration of gingival health in these patients:

1. The encouragement of motivation. There are a number of ways of achieving this and perhaps the most effective is to demonstrate disease in the patient's mouth. The demonstration of periodontal pockets and bleeding, especially if there are healthy sites for comparison, may in most patients give them sufficient interest in the measures needed to restore health.
2. Link the disease to the cause (e.g. dental plaque), again by the demonstration of this in their own mouths. The use of disclosing agents may assist in this part of the process.
3. Provide information on the methods that can be adopted to remove plaque and restore health.
4. Instruct the patient in appropriate methods of oral hygiene.
5. Set realistic targets for the patient's plaque control. The use of an appropriate index for the plaque level and gingival inflammation will be of great assistance in this phase of the treatment.

This is only a broad outline of some appropriate methods of oral hygiene. Further information can be found earlier in this book and in the section on dental health education.

In addition to the advice on oral hygiene, it is also helpful to undertake a professional prophylaxis for patients with gingivitis. This leaves the mouth clean, starts the healing process, and has the effect of reinforcing the patient's home care. The removal of calculus and overhanging margins of restorations makes oral hygiene more effective, and the removal of stains and plaque gives a sparkle to the teeth that all patients appreciate.

It will be necessary to follow up the patient to monitor the effect of your advice, provide feedback and reinforce the motivation. Figure 8.1a and b illustrates the improvement that may be obtained in these patients.

Management of adult periodontitis

Adult type periodontitis is, after chronic gingivitis, the commonest of the periodontal diseases (Figure 8.2). Unlike gingivitis, in which the inflammation is confined to the superficial gingival tissues, periodontitis affects all of the periodontal tissues especially the ligament or membrane. It may be accompanied by a variable amount of gingivitis, which may differ not only from patient to patient, but also from one site to another in the mouth. The characteristics of periodontitis are loss of attachment caused by the apical

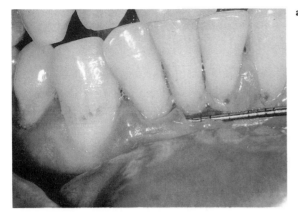

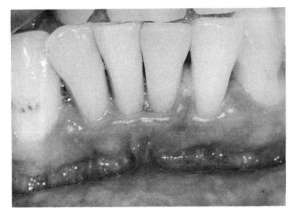

Figure 8.1   Chronic periodontal disease: (a) a patient with inflammatory periodontal disease prior to treatment. The gingiva are loose and oedematous and may be easily reflected from the teeth to reveal subgingival plaque and calculus deposits; (b) the same patient after initial therapy. The gingiva have healed and cannot now be separated from the root surface. The level of plaque deposits is low

migration of the junctional epithelium, which may present as pocketing and/or recession, together with bone loss. In the later stages mobility and drifting of the affected teeth may occur. Other symptoms may include halitosis and pus formation in walls of the pockets, some of which progress to lateral periodontal abscesses.

Adult periodontitis usually occurs in older patients whose tissues respond well to plaque-induced damage and break down slowly over a long period of time. Although there may be periods of rapid breakdown, as with any type of inflammatory disease, generally the increase in probing depths is slow. There may be a large amount of reparative fibrosis in the inflamed gingiva.

The management of all forms of periodontitis is necessarily complex and time consuming and the main principles are as follows:

1. The assessment and diagnosis of the disease. It is the responsibility of the dental surgeon to carry out the necessary screening of patients under their care, to undertake an assessment and to arrive at an appropriate

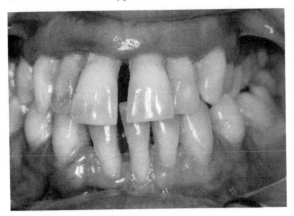

Figure 8.2   Adult periodontitis. There are heavy deposits of plaque, recession has occurred and probing would reveal pocketing. The teeth are mobile and drifting has occurred. Radiographs would show extensive bone loss

treatment plan. The dental hygienist may be involved in the assessment, carrying out many of the investigations such as measuring plaque and gingival levels, as well as periodontal probing depths.

2. Discussion of the findings with the patient to determine their attitudes and expectations. At this stage relief of pain, if present, may be carried out. Decisions on any teeth of hopeless prognosis (i.e. those with practically no supporting bone) should be made at this stage to avoid any misunderstanding about what might be achieved with therapy.

3. Provide the appropriate plaque control including advice on home care measures and the removal of plaque retention factors such as calculus. This part of treatment is often called the 'hygiene phase' or 'cause-related' therapy. Home care would usually involve a subgingival brushing technique, interdental cleansing and, for many patients, the use of disclosing agents where supragingival plaque control measures are suspect. In some patients the use of chemical adjuncts to plaque control may be indicated and this is discussed elsewhere in the book.

4. Following this phase of treatment, a period of time, often 6–12 weeks, is allowed for healing before the tissue response is reassessed and a decision is made on the need for further treatment.

5. The treatment following the hygiene phase will depend upon the healing response. It may include one or more of the following:
   (a) If good healing has been achieved, or if there are signs that healing is occurring, the patient is monitored and where indicated treated to ensure that the tissues return to maintainable health.
   (b) If a healing response is not occurring and the home care is inadequate then the cause should be sought and further advice on oral hygiene provided.
   (c) Where the lack of healing is accompanied by an adequate level of home care, root planing would be carried out as described elsewhere in this text.

6. For the small group of patients who do not respond to the above regimes

it may be necessary for periodontal surgery to be undertaken and this is described later in this chapter.

Management of aggressive periodontal diseases

There are a number of types of periodontal diseases which may be considered to be aggressive inflammatory conditions, either because they occur in younger age groups than adult type periodontitis or because they progress at a more rapid rate, and for this reason they are often termed 'aggressive or progressive disease'. These periodontal diseases may be categorized as:

1. Prepubertal periodontitis.
2. Juvenile periodontitis.
3. Rapidly progressive periodontitis.
4. Refractory periodontitis.

Prepubertal periodontitis

As can be judged from its name, prepubertal periodontitis occurs in children before adolescence (Figure 8.3). The greatest incidence occurs during the eruption of the permanent dentition although the primary teeth are not exempt from its ravages. The occurrence of true pocketing and progressive periodontitis in children is rare and when it occurs is often a sign of a systemic defect, although in some children no underlying predisposing disease can be demonstrated. The diseases that have been identified in sufferers of prepubertal periodontitis include Papillon–Lefevre syndrome, insulin-dependent diabetes, primary or acquired immunodeficiency, leukaemias, hypophosphatasia, histiocytosis X, neutropenia and agranulocytosis.

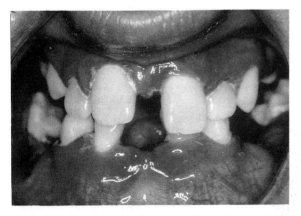

Figure 8.3 Prepubertal periodontitis. The teeth are exfoliating as they erupt. The patient suffers from Papillon–Lefevre syndrome

The characteristics of this disease are not well known, although localized and generalized forms have been described. The gingival inflammation is extremely acute and granulation or proliferation from the active sites may occur, giving rise to gingival epulides of the pyogenic variety. There is often very rapid destruction of alveolar bone and sometimes gingival recession.

Immune system defects including functional defects of peripheral blood leucocytes and monocytes may be found in these patients and a lack of neutrophils has been described in the affected gingival tissues. The patients may also have a history of other problems, including respiratory and middle-ear infections. Little is known about the microbiology of this disease.

Management
The overriding need in these patients is to undertake systemic screening to identify or eliminate any systemic defect. Although in many patients the results may prove negative, the identification of a serious defect in even a small number will justify such an approach. In the others it will be a relief for the child and guardians to learn that the problem is confined to the mouth. The techniques of these investigations and their follow-up is outside the scope of this text, but should include as a very minimum the following tests:

1. Whole blood count and film.
2. Differential white cell count.
3. Serum chemistry, including random serum glucose.
4. Serum folate, iron, vitamin B_{12} and total iron binding capacity.
5. Urine analysis (dip stick) including glucose and protein.

If any of these indices prove positive, referral and further tests would be necessary depending upon the nature of the defect.

The periodontal therapy, although secondary to the general treatment, often proves to be difficult. Patients of this age are a challenge to anyone providing oral hygiene advice and the root surface treatment will need to be undertaken with sympathy and tact. The use of relative analgesia or sometimes general anaesthesia may be necessary if root planing is required. Some success may be obtained by the use of long courses of antibiotics such as tetracycline or chemotherapeutic agents such as metronidazole.

As a general rule these patients will require regular visits of short duration. The most effective therapies are thorough prophylaxis of the active sites with a low abrasive fluoride-containing paste, together with flushing of the pockets with an ultrasonic scaler, making use of the cavitation effect. Oral hygiene should be kept simple and the guardian must be involved in its supervision and monitoring. Scrub brushing will give some subgingival cleaning. Interdental tape, perhaps with a floss holder, must be used interdentally in the affected area. The guardian may also be shown how to flush the lesion with a subgingival irrigator filled with an antiplaque chemical such as chlorhexidine.

The periodontal therapy is often a holding action pending the rectification of the systemic defect, which once controlled will lead to resolution of the periodontal problem.

Juvenile periodontitis

Juvenile periodontitis is an unusual form of periodontitis which occurs around the permanent teeth of adolescents (Figure 8.4a and b). Classically the periodontal lesions occur around the first molars (Figure 8.5) and the incisors although, as with prepubertal periodontitis, localized and generalized forms have been described. The disease has its onset at puberty, although it may present at any time between 11 and 13 years. More females than males are seen with this problem in treatment clinics but epidemiological investigations in the community have shown that the prevalence is equal in both males and females.

The amount of gingival inflammation seen in these patients is frequently low and the oral hygiene may vary from excellent to appalling. In all patients, however, the degree of breakdown is excessive for the amount and duration of the local irritants. There is some evidence that this disease may be subject to remission or burn-out.

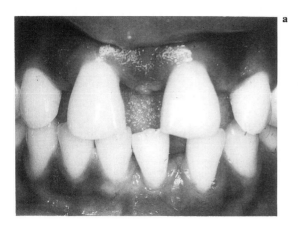

a

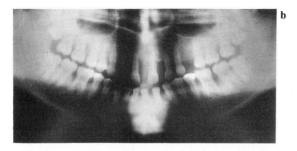

b

Figure 8.4   Juvenile periodontitis in a 19-year-old female: (a) the incisors are mobile and have drifted. Note the good standard of oral hygiene and low levels of superficial inflammation; (b) the orthopantomograph shows severe bone loss in the upper arch and localized loss around the lower first molars

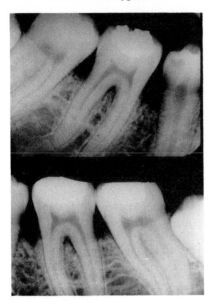

Figure 8.5 Juvenile periodontitis. Early bone loss around first molars and in the furcation areas revealed by radiographs

The defects occur in siblings and the familial distribution is consistent with an autosomal recessive genetic trait. It is thought that all affected individuals probably have functional defects of neutrophils or monocytes. The microbiology has been studied in some depth and two endotoxin-producing organisms *Actinobacillus actinomycetemcomitans* and *Capnocytophaga* have been identified in a large number of these patients. Interestingly these toxins inhibit phagocytic cell function, which may account for the defects seen in the neutrophil and monocyte function.

Management
Although the treatment of these patients follows the general principles laid down for adult type periodontitis, the rapidity of the progression of this condition makes the monitoring much more critical. There are two areas in which management does, however, differ radically. It is now widely accepted that these patients should be treated with tetracycline to eradicate the associated organisms. It is a matter of clinical judgement whether the antibiotic is given immediately the condition is diagnosed, or with root surface treatment. There is some evidence that this condition does not respond well to root planing, and the most optimal result is obtained from a combination of early surgery and tetracycline. The current recommendation for the antibiotic regime is for oxytetracycline 250 mg taken four times a day for 3 weeks, assuming the patient is of average weight. If surgery is combined with this, a replaced flap should be used.

Rapidly progressive periodontitis

This has been recently described in the literature. Typically the sufferers have severe and rapidly advancing lesions (Figure 8.6). There is some disagreement as to when it first occurs although the consensus is that it is usually seen between the ages of 25 and 35 years. The lesions are frequently generalized with all the teeth affected to a greater or lesser degree, without any consistent pattern of destruction. During the active phases the lesions are acutely inflamed and may proliferate to give rise to granulomatous gingival epulides. Some three-quarters of the patients have been shown to have functional defects of neutrophils or monocytes and systemic manifestations including depression, weight loss and general malaise have been reported.

This type of periodontitis has been reported to follow juvenile periodontitis in some patients and is also more commonly seen in sufferers of certain systemic diseases. There is a higher prevalence in individuals with Down's or Chediak–Higashi syndromes and insulin-dependent diabetes.

Management
Again the general principles of the treatment of periodontitis apply to these patients. Recently treatment with tetracycline, metronidazole or a combination of metronidazole and amoxicillin has been advocated, with variable results. The use of a subgingival irrigation with chlorhexidine is often helpful.

Refractory periodontitis

In a small number of sites in some patients the periodontal lesion will remain active, as shown by continued signs of inflammation, pus formation or pocket deepening despite active treatment. Before attempting to retreat and stabilize this type of lesion, it is necessary to stop and consider the reasons

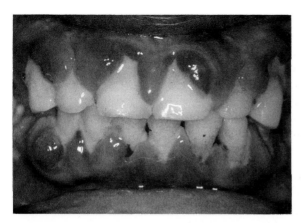

Figure 8.6 Rapidly progressive periodontitis. There is aggressively advancing periodontitis with a florid tissue response

for the failure of the site to heal. The more frequent reasons are, in order of probability:

1. Inadequate oral hygiène.
2. Persistence of root surface deposits.
3. Root surface defects.
4. Inadequate host response.
5. Unidentified systemic factor.

Inadequate oral hygiene may be defined as a level of supragingival dental plaque which is incompatible with marginal periodontal health. This will vary from patient to patient, but the clinical level of residual plaque should be sufficiently low to permit the marginal gingival tissues to be free of visible inflammation. If marginal inflammation persists, then a complex subgingival flora is soon re-established and pocket activity will again occur.

Root surface deposits are always left after treatment but usually the host response is able to cope with a low level of retained irritants, such as dental plaque, calculus and cementum-bound endotoxin. However, it is not always possible to debride the root surface adequately due to difficulties with access, visibility or root contour as shown in Figure 8.7. In general, anterior, single rooted teeth are usually amenable to instrumentation, whilst posterior, multiple rooted teeth with furcation involvements are least likely to be successfully treated.

Root surface defects such as grooves, flutes, gingival pits or enamel projections are seen in some sites with refractory inflammation. The root surface defects prevent complete debridement and inflammation will persist.

Inadequate host response is seen in a small number of individuals who usually have defects involving their polymorphonuclear leucocytes or monocytes. These defects are difficult to detect and impossible to treat. The only factor that can be changed in these unfortunate patients is to reduce the level of plaque deposits even further.

Unidentified systemic factors such as anaemia, diabetes or other similar problems occur in a very small number of patients. Although it is not appropriate to screen all patients with refractory lesions, if multiple sites are

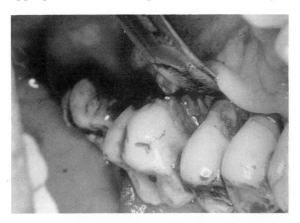

Figure 8.7 Calculus deposits revealed by the raising of a periodontal flap. This calculus has been planed smooth and would be difficult to detect during 'closed' root planing

active, the tissues highly inflamed and the plaque levels low, it is worthwhile for the patient to have a haematological screening including whole blood count, film and serum chemistry.

Management
There are a number of actions that can be taken to stabilize a refractory lesion:

1. Recheck the home care measures.
2. Introduce subgingival irrigation.
3. Repeat the root planing.
4. Prescribe systemic chemotherapeutic agents.
5. Undertake periodontal flap surgery.
6. Continue prolonged frequent professional debridement.

Recheck the home care
The basics of home care have been covered in the section on the control of deposits, but there are some aspects that it is worthwhile to recheck.

Firstly, check that the patient is using a subgingival brushing method. It is important to note that although many methods of brushing, such as the Roll technique, are quite adequate for the healthy patient, they will not cope with the presence of pocketing or gingival swelling. Also ensure that the patient is using a disclosing agent (tablets or liquid) after brushing to monitor residual plaque levels.

The necessity for good daily interdental cleansing must be stressed and insisted upon. Finally, ensure that the environment in which oral hygiene is undertaken is adequate. Good lighting, a mirror – preferably a magnifying one – and a comfortable seat are essential.

Subgingival irrigation
Some studies have shown that the introduction of a chemical antiseptic such as 0.2% chlorhexidine digluconate into the pocket will have an additional depressant effect on the subgingival flora. There are two main ways of introducing the chemical subgingivally: the use of a pulsed water irrigator or by using a syringe with a large blunt needle. The irrigation should be undertaken on a daily basis until the lesion is under control.

Repetition of root planing
It is worthwhile repeating the root planing on a tooth adjacent to an active site on at least two occasions with a period of at least 3–6 months in between. It must be remembered that it may take up to 6 months for the full effects of root planing to be achieved. Root planing should include the use of an ultrasonic or sonic scaler, as the flushing effect will reduce both the level of subgingival microbes and cementum-bound endotoxin.

The root planing may be combined with chemical irrigation or the use of systemic chemotherapeutic agents.

Systemic chemotherapeutic agents
The use of systemic agents such as amoxicillin, tetracycline, metronidazole and Septrin may in some cases produce dramatic improvements, provided

they are combined with mechanical root surface treatment in the form of root planing or flap surgery.

Tetracycline is the most popular antibiotic and is used in a dosage of 250 mg four times a day for 2–3 weeks for an average adult. Metronidazole is also a useful agent when 200 mg are taken three times a day for 1–2 weeks. Recently a regime combining both metronidazole and amoxicillin for 7 days has been described, with significant improvements noted.

Septrin, which is a combination of a folic acid inhibitor and a sulphonamide (trimethoprim and sulphamethoxazole) is also a useful broad spectrum chemotherapeutic agent that has a use in the treatment of refractory cases. An appropriate dosage would be two tablets twice daily for 4 weeks.

Periodontal flap surgery

For those sites which persist despite the previous treatment and when the home care is considered adequate, the raising of a periodontal flap is necessary to permit access to the root surface for instrumentation. The commonest procedure undertaken is the replaced flap, often called the modified Widman procedure. It is worthwhile to use the access gained by this procedure to polish the root surface using a sterile bristle brush with a biocompatible abrasive such as calcium hydroxide. Polishing a root surface has recently been shown to be the most effective way of reducing the surface cementum-bound endotoxin.

Professional debridement

Sometimes, when the lesions will not stabilize, it is necessary to undertake repeated professional debridement of the active pockets, especially with the sonic or ultrasonic scaler. This will be sufficient in many patients to prevent extension of the lesions with the problems of further loss of attachment.

However, despite carrying out all these procedures to a high level, some sites do progress and ultimately may lead to loss of the tooth.

Chapter 9

Acute periodontal disorders

The majority of acute periodontal problems are superimposed upon an underlying chronic inflammatory condition and may present a considerable challenge in terms of the management of the hygiene problems. A good example of this is acute necrotizing gingivitis, which is most frequently seen in patients who are suffering from chronic gingivitis or periodontitis. Home care may be difficult because of gingival soreness and root surface treatment similarly hindered.

However, some acute problems such as those relating to trauma may arise in relatively healthy mouths. Traditionally, acute periodontal disorders are divided into those primarily affecting the gingiva and those affecting the periodontal ligament. All forms of acute gingivitis have the common signs of erythema, oedematous swelling and will be sore. Other signs and symptoms will depend upon the underlying causes, as discussed below.

Acute traumatic gingivitis

This condition may be caused by physical, thermal or chemical factors. Diagnosis will usually be apparent from the history, together with the appearance of the lesions.

Physical causes include toothbrush trauma, especially when a new brush has recently been purchased and damage from foreign bodies inserted into the mouth, an activity particularly common in children. One type of damage may be caused deliberately by the patient – a condition termed 'gingivitis artefacta'. When this condition is associated with a psychiatric disorder it is termed 'gingivitis artefacta major' and when it is an innocent habit it may be termed 'minor'. Despite its innocent background severe damage may be caused to the gingiva, even leading to tooth loss, as shown in Figure 9.1. This problem is particularly seen in young children.

Other causes of acute traumatic gingivitis are damage from hard food and iatrogenic damage from dental treatment. Many dental procedures have the ability to cause transient gingivitis. These include cavity preparation adjacent to the gingiva and gingival abrasion by brushes and burs.

In all such situations the gingiva will be eroded to some degree, often with a ragged margin with visible tags of damaged epithelium. Long-standing

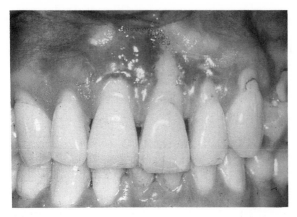

Figure 9.1 Gingivitis artefacta. The labial gingiva has been traumatically removed by finger scratching. The patient 'liked' the feeling of scratching the gingiva

cases will have a surrounding area of keratosis where the stimulus has been less acute.

Thermal causes are principally caused by eating hot food. The classic history of hot, melted cheese on French onion soup or fondues sticking to and burning the gingiva is well known. Dental cautery or overheated ultrasonic scalers may produce similar damage. The history of the condition will usually be characteristic.

Chemical trauma may be caused by a number of substances. Burns caused by the application of aspirin to the gingiva alongside a tooth that is a source of pain, in the belief that this will have a local or topical effect, are still occasionally seen (Figure 3.7). Iatrogenic chemical burns have increased since the advent of etch retained composites. The etchant contains approximately 50% phosphoric acid and if this is allowed to run down into the gingiva will cause a brisk acute gingivitis. As well as a relevant history, the early chemical lesion will have a white covering where the epithelium has been damaged but this is rapidly lost to leave a tender area of acute gingivitis.

Management

The first step in the management of patients with acute traumatic forms of gingivitis is to identify the cause. Some patients may not admit to a damaging habit and food trauma may not be noticed at the time, especially if the meal has been accompanied by alcohol. Once the cause has been identified, treatment is directed towards reassuring the sufferer and providing palliative measures such as lignocaine gel to ease the pain and antiseptic mouthwashes to decrease the duration of secondary infection. An alternative mouthwash, particularly if a thermal burn is suspected, is benzydamine hydrochloride, which will decrease soreness considerably. If the condition is being aggravated by aggressive brushing, it might be advisable for the patient to stop brushing for a period and rely on the use of a chemical antiplaque agent. This will allow keratinization of the abraded gingiva to occur, prior to brushing being resumed. Some areas may be amenable to coverage with periodontal dressings or adhesive patches to facilitate healing and prevent further damage.

Acute non-specific gingivitis

This condition is most commonly seen as an acute exacerbation of pre-existing chronic gingivitis (Figure 9.2). The diagnosis is made by excluding other causes of acute gingivitis including acute necrotizing and herpetic gingivitis. It may be associated with a lowering of host resistance, such as occurs with systemic illnesses. There may also be local causes such as lack of lip seal in the upper incisor area or mouth breathing which may cause palatal acute gingivitis.

Management

Often, although there is no practical treatment of the precipitating cause, careful oral hygiene together with scaling and polishing will allow recovery to occur. Where the soreness of the condition makes oral hygiene difficult, then the use of chemical methods of plaque control is indicated.

Acute hypersensitivity reactions

Hypersensitivity reactions to the constituents of toothpastes and occasionally cosmetics are sometimes seen as an 'allergic gingivitis' (Figure 9.3). The

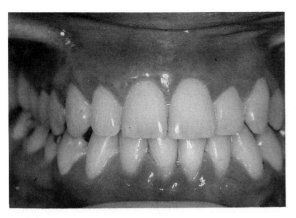

Figure 9.2 Acute non-specific gingivitis. The gingivae are red and sore. This is an exacerbation of the underlying gingivitis

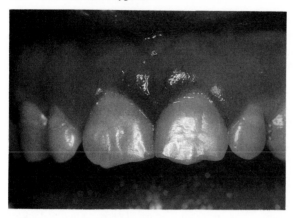

Figure 9.3 Acute hypersensitivity reaction to a new toothpaste. The gingiva returned to normal after discontinuing use of the toothpaste, and returned following the subsequent reuse

symptoms reported may vary considerably but a common feature is a widespread diffuse granular gingivitis involving the full width of the attached gingiva. Other features may include oral ulceration, glossitis and cheilitis. The commonest hypersensitivity reaction is to the cinnamonaldehyde constituent of toothpastes. This flavouring is currently used in tartar control toothpastes to hide the unpleasant taste of the pyrophosphate active agent. The histological features of gingival biopsies are generally non-specific although the presence of a plasma cell infiltration may sometimes be seen.

Management

An important principle in the treatment of these patients is not to expose them to further chemicals to which they may react. The urge to use a chemical antiplaque agent should be avoided and the patient should be reassured and the toothpaste changed to allow healing to occur.

Acute necrotizing gingivitis

This is an acute gingivitis characterized by necrotizing interdental ulcers which rapidly spread to the other areas of the gingiva. Characteristically the ulcers are covered by a yellowish pseudomembrane which is composed of sloughed epithelial cells, polymorphs, fusiforms and spirochaetes in a fibrinous exudate. The condition is usually very painful and the gingiva are very sore to touch and bleed easily on manipulation.

There is a characteristic halitosis and the sufferer may report spontaneous haemorrhage from the ulcers (Figure 9.4). Systemically there may be swelling and tenderness of the regional lymph nodes together with fever and malaise. Although the condition starts as an acute condition it often subsides into a chronic state which is identical to adult type periodontitis, except for the presence of typical tissue deformities. This state has been termed chronic necrotizing gingivitis (Lindhe, 1989), although the American Academy of

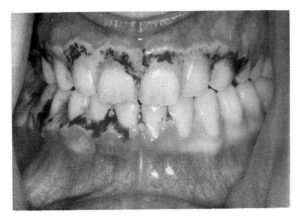

Figure 9.4   Acute necrotizing gingivitis. The gingiva are ulcerated and bleeding spontaneously

Periodontology has recently adopted the term acute necrotizing *periodontitis*, which is more logical in view of the loss of attachment that is an invariable consequence of this stage of the disorder.

The aetiology of the condition is unclear but certain common predisposing conditions may be observed. The patient, who is frequently aged between 18 and 30 years, usually has a pre-existing inflammatory periodontal disorder, either gingivitis or periodontitis, and often is a smoker. There may be a history of a recent systemic illness such as the common cold which lowers the tissue resistance, or the disease may follow a stressful episode in the patient's life such as bereavement, divorce or redundancy. Recently the disease has been found to have a high occurrence in HIV infected individuals.

The microbiology of the condition is interesting. Vincent (1898) first described the *fusospirochaetal complex* consisting of the micro-organisms, *Bacillus fusiformis* and *Borrelia vincentii*. Since that time a variety of other organisms have been shown to be usually present including *Vibrio*, *Bacteroides* and *Selenomonas* species. The part played by these organisms in the development of the condition is unclear.

Management

The management of the sufferers from acute necrotizing gingivitis is based on recognition of the predisposing factors. In view of the relationship to stress and the need for careful home care to prevent recurrence, a very careful explanation of the problem together with the treatment needed should be provided to the patient. Advice should be given on the avoidance of smoking and the need for an adequate diet. The initial acute phase should be treated by careful debridement of the lesions with the spray from an ultrasonic scaler. Advice on home care should include the advice to purchase a new toothbrush. Although colonization of the toothbrush bristles by the organisms involved in the condition is a theoretical possibility, the main reason for the advice is to ensure that an adequate brush is used.

Many periodontists would prescribe the drug metronidazole (Flagyl), 200 mg, taken three times a day with meals for 3 days. This chemotherapeutic agent is very effective against the Gram-negative organisms involved. However, there are some worries about its teratogenic potential and its use in pregnancy is contraindicated. Penicillin is a safe and effective alternative.

It will be necessary to follow up the patient as relapse and recurrence is common. As the condition usually occurs in patients with a pre-existing inflammatory periodontal condition, this will require treatment once the acute phase is under control. In some patients gingival deformities caused by the interdental ulceration will require surgical correction, either by gingivoplasty or flap surgery.

HIV-associated gingivitis

Recently an acute form of gingivitis has been described which is seen in sufferers from Acquired Immune Deficiency Syndrome (AIDS) and has been categorized as a definitive form of gingivitis. It is most probable that these conditions are only an exaggerated or unusual response to dental plaque due to the immune deficits that occur in these patients.

The commonest symptom is an intense marginal gingivitis in a patient who has been diagnosed as infected with the Human Immunodeficiency Virus (HIV). In the more severe cases, there may be ulceration similar to that seen in acute necrotizing ulcerative gingivitis.

Management

The primary treatment in these patients is directed towards coping with the HIV infection. The oral lesions should always be reported to the consulting physician as they may indicate the development of AIDS in an HIV sufferer. The oral lesions should be sampled with a smear for candidal infection as this is often present and may cause an acute form of gingivitis. Assuming that no unusual organisms are found, reinforcing the oral hygiene, together with chemical plaque control by using an 0.2% chlorhexidine gluconate mouthrinse, will help to control the problem.

Acute herpetic gingivostomatitis

The oral cavity may be involved in infection with herpes simplex viruses types I and II. Infection with type I usually occurs in childhood, but because infection is increasingly avoided in childhood it is becoming more common in both adolescents and adults (Figure 9.5). Type II infection, which is usually sexually transmitted, is more commonly seen in adults. Clinically both types have similar oral manifestations. The oral signs are soreness of the oral mucosa, with small vesicles which form and rapidly burst to form ulcers surrounded by a bright red halo. There may also be a concomitant marginal herpetic gingivitis. Systemically there is often malaise, fever and

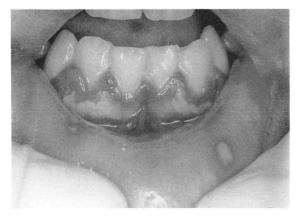

Figure 9.5   Acute herpetic gingivostomatitis. The gingiva is erythematous and widespread ulceration is present

lymphadenitis. Children will be irritable, salivate excessively and may have difficulty in eating. Dehydration may occur within a short period of time.

Management

Diagnosis is made on clinical grounds backed up by laboratory tests such as immunofluoresence or a rising antibody titre. The most important aspect of management is to correct any fluid imbalance by encouraging fluid intake and advise bed rest. Food should be soft and cold items may be soothing. This is one of the few occasions when the clinician may recommend ice cream with no sense of guilt.

The use of a 0.2% chlorhexidine gluconate mouthrinse will help to reduce the severity of secondary infection in the oral lesions. In the older patient the use of benzocaine lozenges or lignocaine viscous paint will help to reduce discomfort during eating. Paracetamol or aspirin can also be recommended to reduce discomfort and lower temperature and promethazine elixir will act as a sedative and allow sleep in the younger child.

When there are severe systemic symptoms acyclovir may be taken either as tablets or as an elixir. The cream presentation is also useful in treating the problems of herpes labialis.

Acute periodontal abscess

A periodontal abscess occurs when pus collects in the connective tissue wall of a pocket (Figure 9.6). It is important to distinguish this from a periapical abscess caused by a non-vital tooth, and to emphasize this distinction the term *lateral* periodontal abscess is often used. The differential diagnosis may be made based on the history, the clinical examination, vitality tests and appropriate radiographs.

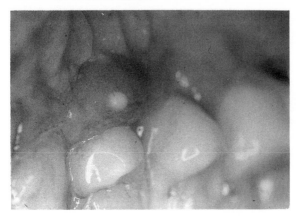

Figure 9.6   Acute periodontal abscess. Pus is pointing through the palatal mucosa and can also be expressed through the pocket

It is unusual for a periodontal abscess to occur in the absence of severe periodontitis, although it may be initiated by acute trauma. The precipitating causes are not clearly understood and it is quite possible that they may vary from patient to patient. Among the factors that have been implicated are:

1. Entry of organisms into the connective tissues adjacent to the periodontal pocket, which has been shown to occur in deep periodontal lesions.
2. The forcing of plaque, calculus and other irritant debris through the pocket lining during scaling and root planing procedures.
3. Impaction of foreign bodies into the periodontal pocket. This is often quoted as a cause of the problem but the authors have never seen a periodontal abscess associated with this type of damage.
4. Blockage of a pocket with obstruction of drainage. Although this is a possible cause, the majority of abscesses seen are draining through the pocket on presentation.
5. Reduction of host resistance as seen in some conditions such as diabetes, which are associated with frequent periodontal abscesses.

The abscess may present as a localized swelling with erythema of the overlying mucosa. The tooth may be tender to biting or percussion, and the patient may complain of throbbing which is relieved by pressure. The swelling is frequently, but not invariably, fluctuant. There may be systemic symptoms, such as lymphadenitis of the local lymph nodes, as well as raised temperature. This is more common when the condition is acute, but once drainage has been achieved the abscess becomes chronic with a lessening of symptoms.

Management

The initial problem is managed by establishing drainage, so the first joint decision to be made by the operator and patient is whether this should be achieved by extracting the tooth.

If it is decided to attempt to save the tooth, initial drainage may be obtained by scaling and root planing the lesion. Should this not relieve the pressure then a fluctuant lesion can be incised at its most dependent point or by raising a small flap to expose the defect and allow effective debridement. Any local anaesthesia used must not be placed into the inflamed area.

The patient should be advised to use hot salt water mouthrinses during the healing period. Once the lesion has settled further, root planing or surgery may be required to encourage healing. This type of lesion will require careful, long-term follow-up to ensure that recurrence does not occur.

HIV-associated periodontitis

Recently an acute form of periodontitis been described in sufferers from Acquired Immune Deficiency Syndrome (AIDS) and categorized as a definitive form of periodontitis. It is thought that the depression of the immune system that occurs in sufferers from AIDS allows severe forms of periodontitis to occur (Figure 9.7).

The symptoms vary widely from acute necrotizing gingivitis-type infection to widespread ulceration with soft tissue and bony exposure and necrosis, and exfoliation of the teeth in severe cases.

Management

The primary treatment in these patients is directed towards treating the HIV infection. A smear for candidal infection should be taken as this is common in AIDS sufferers. The treatment should be conservative, with use of 0.2% chlorhexidine gluconate mouthrinse, together with antibiotics to control the oral infection.

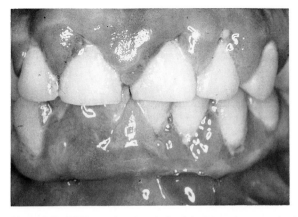

Figure 9.7 HIV-associated periodontitis. There is aggressive breakdown of the periodontal tissues with marginal ulceration and severe erythema

Chapter 10

Other preventive and therapeutic procedures

Control of cross infection

Transmission of disease in the clinical environment may occur in a variety of ways. After initial contact with the skin of infected blood, saliva or respiratory secretions, organisms may penetrate the surface via a cut or skin abrasion. Alternatively, access to the patient's or clinician's bloodstream can follow a stab injury involving a contaminated needle or item of equipment. At times infection can occur after ingestion of organisms or following direct penetration of a mucous surface.

The close proximity of dental health care personnel to patients puts both at particular risk from inhalation of infected aerosols. Such aerosols may be produced by coughing and sneezing but are also associated with dental procedures and are enhanced considerably by some of the equipment used in dental practice. It has been shown that handpieces, triple syringes, ultrasonic scalers and even toothbrushing instruction are all responsible for producing significant aerosols. To protect the moist mucosal surfaces at risk from aerosol infection a facemask and spectacles should be worn. Protective spectacles are essential for the operator, whose eyes are particularly at risk from flying particles of infected calculus, filling material, tooth tissue and blood, and should also be worn by patients during any procedures during which there is danger of eye damage especially when being treated in the supine position.

To further reduce the risks of infection by contact or droplet spread from coughing and sneezing, facemasks and latex gloves should also be worn by ancillary members of the dental team – these help provide both the clinician and patient with a basic means of infection control.

The clinician can not only be the original source of infection but can also be the vehicle for transmission between patients. In most cases of cross-infection the source of the causative organism is difficult to establish and this, in conjunction with the possibility that some patients may be asymptomatic carriers of disease, emphasizes the importance of following a strict programme of asepsis before, during and after each patient visit.

Destruction of micro-organisms

While most vegetative forms of micro-organism can be easily killed, many are capable of entering a spore phase which is highly resistant to heat and desiccation. In this form they can survive, for a limited time, even the most adverse conditions and for this reason immersion of instruments in boiling water can no longer be justified as a means of cross-infection control.

Greater efforts are required if contamination of instruments with blood or saliva has occurred. When coated with dried proteinaceous deposits the ability of bacteria and viruses to survive is enhanced. Thorough cleaning of instruments, preferably by means of an ultrasonic cleanser, is the essential first stage before starting any disinfection or sterilization routine.

Disinfection
Chemical disinfectants are formulated to kill pathogenic micro-organisms but may not kill all the micro-organisms present. They are used principally to clean operating surfaces and some equipment in the clinical environment. Their use does not guarantee sterility, and their application in infection control procedures must always be assessed critically. Their clinical effectiveness is difficult to quantify because simple, reliable tests have not yet been developed which provide an objective confirmation of sterility in the conditions under which they are used. The chemical solutions which are considered most effective and which appear suitable for surfaces, instruments and items such as impressions that cannot be heat sterilized are included in Table 10.1.

Sterilization
This is a process which results in destruction of all micro-organisms and is normally achieved in the surgery by heat, and all dental practices must possess an effective means of sterilizing instruments that are used in the mouth. At present the most popular and most time-efficient method is the autoclave which produces its effect by means of superheated steam. The hot air oven is reserved for specific functions such as sterilization of burs and reamers. In North America alternative sterilizing techniques are available such as chemical vapour sterilization ('Chemiclave'), whereby a mixture of chemicals (ethyl alcohol, isopropyl alcohol, formaldehyde, acetone and

Table 10.1   The commoner chemical disinfectants used in dentistry and their uses

Type	Use
Glutaraldehyde	Instruments that cannot be autoclaved and impressions. Valuable for maintaining sterility of instruments
Iodophors	Hard surfaces and hands
Hexachloraphene	Hands
Alcohol/chlorhexidine	Surfaces and impressions

butanone) is heated to 127°C at 210 kPa for 30 min in equipment similar to an autoclave. The advantage of this system is that rusting is not produced and it is faster than using a hot air oven. Irradiation is one of the large-scale techniques used in industry to sterilize disposable goods (e.g. latex gloves, sutures and needles) for clinical use. The alternative – use of ethylene oxide gas – is not used in the surgery but is more commonly employed in the sterilization departments of larger hospitals.

Autoclave

This is the most popular and quickest method of sterilising dental instruments. Autoclaves can operate effectively at a temperature of 134°C, when the contents are maintained for 3 min at a pressure of 210 kPa or at 121°C when 15 min at 105 kPa is required. Under either of these conditions all forms of micro-organisms will be destroyed. It is important that all instruments to be sterilized come into contact with the superheated steam produced during the operating cycle, and therefore all instruments must be cleaned free of debris, rust or scale beforehand. Instrument bags (if used), or instrument trays should not be so tightly packed that steam access is restricted and sterilization incomplete. At the end of the operating cycle, instruments should be allowed to cool gradually. The efficiency of the operating cycle may be confirmed by including in with the instrument load a paper test strip (Albert Browne Ltd, Leicester) containing a chemical which changes colour on reaching the appropriate temperature. This test does not confirm, however, that all micro-organisms are killed.

Hot air oven

This equipment achieves its effect by dry heat at a temperature of 160°C, which is maintained for 1 h. It is suitable for glass and metal items – particularly dental burs – because it does not dull their cutting edges. It is efficient provided that the load is adequately penetrated by the hot air, and care must be taken to ensure that this takes place. Fans ensure that the interior reaches a uniform temperature, and ideally there should be a time lock to ensure effective operation. The main disadvantage is the length of the operating cycle which limits its popularity in busy dental practices.

Surgery hygiene

General cleanliness and waste disposal

Control of micro-organisms in the dental surgery begins with general cleanliness. This involves the physical removal of dust and dirt from floors, walls, furniture and equipment. It should be undertaken each day after the last patient has left. As a minimum standard the clinical environment should be kept as clean as a well cared for home, so that dust is not allowed to collect on horizontal surfaces, and finger prints do not remain on smooth surfaces or on the operating light lens.

Clinical waste should be kept in a suitable container out of sight until disposed of in the correct manner. Omissions and untidiness reflect not only a lack of attention to detail, but will also indicate to the patient the operator's attitude to standards of hygiene in general. 'Sharps' are placed in a marked container for suitable disposal afterwards.

Zoning in the clinical environment
To speed up the process of disinfecting the clinical area while continuing to treat patients, a system of zoning has been recommended. This involves marking with adhesive tape the edges of the areas that become contaminated during patient treatment, and restricting contact of hands, instruments or equipment to those areas. The surfaces to be zoned include the bracket table, the handpieces and triple syringe together with their rests, operating light handles, operating switches on the dental chair and unit, aspirator connectors together with rinsing bowl, and a side surface where soiled articles may be placed until they can be cleaned after the patient has left (Figure 10.1). After each patient has gone, and prior to the arrival of the next, these particular areas may be thoroughly disinfected using an alcohol-based spray (e.g. Dispray, Stuart Pharmaceuticals), or if there is a blood spillage, a 1.0% chlorine-based solution on a disposable paper towel. The main advantage of zoning is to reduce the number of areas contaminated during treatment and make disinfection procedures between patients more streamlined. Zoning in the clinical area is shown in Figure 10.1.

Procedures to follow in practice
Because cross-infection control is so important it is desirable to be familiar with and adopt certain basic routines in clinical practice. These can be summarized as follows.

Preparatory
1. All clinical staff should be vaccinated against hepatitis B.
2. A complete medical history should be taken from all patients.

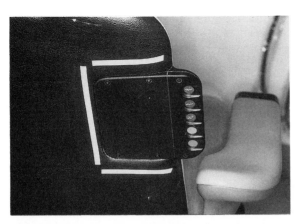

Figure 10.1   An example of zoning in practice with tape outlining an area to be cleaned after each patient. All other 'at risk' areas will be similarly outlined

During treatment
1. Wear gloves, masks and spectacles routinely.
2. Use disposable equipment once only.
3. Use disposable covers or sterilizable trays on surfaces.
4. Beware of needlestick injuries and use a protective device when re-sheathing or disposing of needles.
5. Dry your hands on disposable paper towels.

After treatment
1. After the patient has left, wipe all zoned surfaces with alcohol spray even if they appear clean. Disinfect all contaminated surfaces with 1.0% hypochlorite or 2.0% glutaraldehyde solution. If blood is present, clean with a disposable cloth and 1.0% hypochlorite or 2.0% glutaraldehyde if metal is present.
2. Dispose of waste in an appropriate way:
   (a) Sharps to be placed in a rigid container;
   (b) Other items in sealable plastic bags;
   (c) Arrange for incineration at the end of the day.
3. Clean all instruments thoroughly before sterilization.
4. Use an autoclave cycle of 134°C at 210 kPa for 3 min for sterilizing instruments.
5. Autoclave all instruments including handpieces. Only if unavoidable, use 2.0% glutaraldehyde for 1 h, scrub instruments and soak for a further 3 h.
6. After the last patient, flush the aspirator with 2.0% glutaraldehyde solution and leave overnight.
7. Launder operating gowns on a hot wash programme, 90°C for 10 min.

Care of the high risk patient

Patients known to be hepatitis B or HIV positive may need dental care and can be treated safely in the dental surgery if the above routines are followed. There is no reason for dental care to be refused unless the clinician is immunocompromised or pregnant. To reduce the possibility of the immuno-compromised patient being infected by the operator or other patients, further precautions can be taken:

1. Arrange the appointment for the end of the day so that the patient does not have to wait in a crowded room.
2. Protect essential working surfaces and equipment controls such as chair switches, operating light controls and triple syringe with cling film or plastic bags.
3. Wear a double pair of latex gloves.
4. Use disposable equipment wherever possible.
5. Try to avoid aerosol effects wherever possible.

Concluding comments

Pens and pencils are often overlooked as sources of infection and should be wiped over with disinfectant after each patient. The clinician must keep jewellery to a minimum if worn at all. Ideally latex gloves should be changed between each patient, but washing gloves between each patient with an iodine-based surgical scrub is an acceptable alternative. However, should the gloves become torn or perforated they must be discarded and new ones worn.

Infection control in dental practice should receive a high level of priority and a regular routine established and adopted during and after each patient's treatment. This will take time initially but with experience the time required will decrease and a safe working environment can be maintained.

Moisture control

All the operative work done by a clinician is best performed under dry conditions. Blood and moisture obscure the clear visibility needed for accurate application of instruments. Any form of contamination of the teeth will prevent adhesion when fissure sealants are applied and traces of water and saliva prevent the effective application of desensitizing agents. From the point of view of the patient's comfort the collection of large quantities of fluid in the mouth is not only distressing but can cause involuntary swallowing at inconvenient times. Although atropine is used in general anaesthetic practice, control of saliva flow by drugs is very rarely indicated for dental purposes and in any case has no effect on the other liquid contaminants, namely blood and external water. Consequently, while local cleaning and drying of teeth is easily achieved by use of a triple syringe, the subsequent permanent removal of debris, blood, saliva and water from the operating site has to be accomplished by some mechanical means.

Control of bleeding

When dealing with inflamed tissues some bleeding will inevitably occur. Usually this haemorrhage is capillary in origin, transient and easily removed from the site of operation. When bleeding is heavier and more prolonged, further action is required to secure good visibility and prevent the patient becoming concerned. The best way to control gingival bleeding is by applying pressure to the bleeding site by means of a damp swab. A piece of gauze is rolled up and dampened with water (wetted and wrung out). Controversy exists whether cold or hot water is better – both work well.

The swab must be applied firmly to the bleeding surface for 60 s and repeated until effective. A dry swab is contraindicated – if used it will adhere to the delicate bleeding surfaces and cause further damage when it is removed.

Control of saliva and water

Saliva and water from the triple syringe are removed either by absorption into a suitable material or by aspiration. For much of their work hygienists will need only a simple type of low-volume saliva ejector, improving its effectiveness, as necessary, by adjusting the patient's posture. For other forms of treatment, like desensitization of teeth, polishing restorations or application of fissure sealants, absorption methods or high volume aspiration will be essential. In general the more efficient the method the more intrusive it is and the more likely it is that the patients will find it objectionable. This is particularly the case with children and, before attempting their treatment, all who work in the mouth should be well skilled in the simpler methods of moisture control.

Patient posture and saliva control
For their efficient use, saliva control devices have to be placed where saliva collects and the site of collection is influenced by the anatomical sites at which saliva enters the mouth, gravity, and patient posture. After penetrating the buccinator and the mucosa of the cheek, the ducts of the parotid glands enter the mouth opposite the upper first molar teeth. In an upright patient, parotid saliva flows down the mucosal surfaces of the cheeks to the floor of the mouth where it mixes with the secretion from the submandibular glands which has entered the mouth through the orifices of the submandibular ducts in the midline behind the incisor teeth, and with the secretion of the sublingual glands which has entered the floor of the mouth through numerous small openings. Accumulation of excess saliva is then prevented by reflex swallowing.

Modern dental treatment often takes place with the operator seated and the patient lying in the supine position. It follows that normal flow is altered and, under the influence of gravity, saliva pools at the back of the mouth. Low volume saliva ejectors are not designed to remove saliva from the back of the mouth and although access and visibility of the front teeth will remain good for a time, when treatment is prolonged or when unobstructed visibility of the lower posterior teeth is required, a high volume aspirator is essential. In those few cases where patients are unable to accept the presence of an aspirator and sight of the posterior teeth is impaired, improved visibility may be achieved by uprighting the patient in the chair. Saliva then pools around the lower incisor teeth and can be removed with a low volume saliva ejector.

Absorption methods
The most popular method of saliva removal is by absorption with cotton wool rolls. They are available in a variety of sizes but their effectiveness depends on accurate placement and a knowledge of the sites at which saliva enters the mouth. When isolating mandibular posterior teeth, rolls are first placed in the buccal and lingual sulci (Figure 10.2). For the roll in the lingual sulcus to displace the tongue and reach the floor of the mouth the patient first protrudes the tongue. The roll is placed in position and will then be carried into the depth of the lingual sulcus when the tongue is retruded. To prevent saliva from the parotid gland contaminating the site, a further roll is placed in the upper buccal sulcus in the first molar region, over the entrance of the parotid duct into the mouth (Figure 10.3). In the case of a restless patient who finds difficulty leaving cotton wool rolls in place, a special metal or

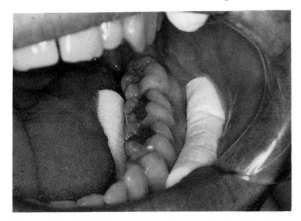

Figure 10.2   Initial placement of cotton wool rolls in buccal and lingual sulcus for isolation of lower posterior teeth

plastic clamp can be applied to a molar tooth with rubber dam forceps. The clamp has a flange on either side to retain a cotton wool roll.

Isolation of lower anterior teeth is carried out in a similar way. A roll is placed first in the lingual sulcus over the ducts of the submandibular salivary glands, with smaller rolls being placed in the labial sulcus.

Gravity ensures that the upper teeth are easier to maintain dry. Rolls need to be placed in the buccal or labial sulcus only. Larger rolls are placed posteriorly where the sulcus is more capacious and smaller rolls anteriorly.

When a dry roll adheres to the dried mucosa, removal is sometimes difficult. If a roll proves difficult or painful to remove it should be saturated with water by means of the triple syringe.

A cotton wool roll can only absorb, at the most, its own volume of saliva and hence the available time for which the operating site remains dry is limited to a few minutes – less if the patient salivates profusely. The time for working in the mouth is further reduced because salivation is stimulated by the presence of foreign bodies such as cotton wool rolls. Newer types of absorbent agent which maintain dry conditions for longer have therefore

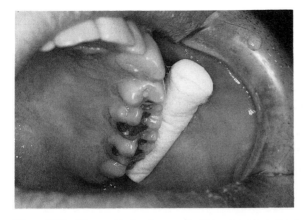

Figure 10.3   Placement of cotton wool roll in upper buccal sulcus over parotid duct

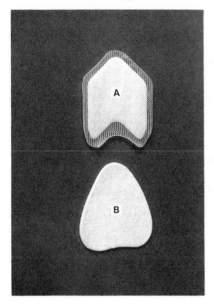

Figure 10.4 Two types of recently developed moisture control device: (A) Dri-Tip; (B) Dri-Guard

been developed (Figure 10.4). One, Dri-Guard (Virilium Co Ltd, Watford), consists of a heart-shaped pad of cellulose fibres. The pad is placed against the cheek in the buccal sulcus where it absorbs parotid saliva. In young patients it also acts as a restraint, warning them by its pressure when they are closing their mouth. An alternative, Dri-Tip (Virilium Co Ltd, Watford), comprises a thin polythene envelope with tea-bag type perforations on one side only. It, too, is placed in the buccal sulcus with the perforated surface next to the cheek. Saliva penetrates the perforations and is absorbed by a central core of hydrogel which can swell to many times its original volume (Figure 10.5). These newer methods can also be supplemented with cotton wool rolls in the lingual sulcus.

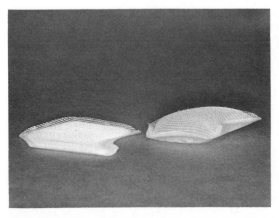

Figure 10.5 Increase in volume shown by saturated Dri-tip

Aspiration

Low volume and high volume aspirators are available. The low volume type is the simple saliva ejector which is available in a variety of designs (Figure 10.6). The least complex is a plastic tube which can be bent to any required shape, but is normally angled so that the tip lies behind the lower incisors over the entrance of the submandibular ducts. The tube contains a wire stiffener which ensures that it remains conformed to the desired shape. Other popular types take the form of a metal flange fitting into the lingual sulcus, or alternatively a plastic flange can be fitted to the tube type. When present, the flange protects the tongue from injury by rotating or sharp instruments. Some forms of saliva ejector also possess a support which fits outside the mouth under the chin and serves to retain the device without the active participation of the patient.

When dealing with children a form of saliva ejector which is sometimes useful consists of a perforated plastic tube rolled up to fit in the lingual sulcus. The flexible material adapts easily to the sulcus and is better accepted than more rigid forms. After rolling up to form a disc, its shape then allows it to act as a form of tongue guard.

While low volume aspiration is satisfactory for most purposes, high volume aspiration becomes necessary when attempting to dry surfaces adequately for purposes of adhesion or when controlling water sprays from the ultrasonic scaler or triple syringe, especially if the 'washed field' technique is being used. In addition, when treating patients in the supine position saliva collects at the back of the mouth unless removed by high volume aspiration. For optimum efficiency the aspirator should be manipulated by an assistant. Placing the tip of the aspirator requires skill. The normal 'rest' position is in the upper molar regions but when using the triple syringe or ultrasonic scaler, or when instrumenting bleeding tissues, close proximity to the site of operation is essential. At no time should the tip of the aspirator come into contact with the patient's soft palate otherwise reflex retching or swallowing might be initiated.

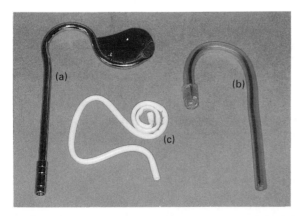

Figure 10.6 Three types of simple low-volume aspirator tip: (a) pre-formed flanged metal saliva ejector; (b) conformable plastic tube with metal wire strengthener; (c) perforated, conformable paper tube

Rubber dam
This method is ideal for ensuring a dry field when applying fissure sealants. In the UK at present its use is restricted to dentists. Use of rubber dam is dealt with in Chapter 13.

Post-surgical maintenance

Immediately following periodontal or flap surgery the patient will either have a periodontal dressing placed or the wound will be closed with sutures. While oral hygiene in the remainder of the mouth can be maintained by routine measures, the presence of a periodontal dressing or 'pack' prevents the beneficial action of normal home care and limits the effectiveness of antiseptic mouthrinses.

Where a pack has been placed the patient should be instructed to avoid chewing sticky foods at the surgical site and to remove accumulated debris by careful rinsing. The patient must also be encouraged to maintain the health of the remainder of the mouth by the usual oral hygiene regime. If sutures and no pack have been used, an antiseptic mouthwash such as 0.2% chlorhexidine gluconate may be prescribed for use twice a day to keep the area plaque-free. A soft brush can be used on the teeth, but interdental cleansing in the surgical area is not to be advised.

Following the removal of a pack or sutures the teeth should be polished with a soft rubber cup, prophy point and a fluoride-containing prophylaxis paste. It is important to maintain professional cleaning on a regular basis for up to 2 months following surgery, because it has been shown that preventing mature plaque deposits reforming improves the healing of the periodontal tissues. It may also be necessary to apply a topical desensitizing agent if exposed root dentine proves sufficiently painful to inhibit home oral hygiene measures.

It is often useful to continue use of an antiseptic mouthwash for at least 2 months following periodontal flap surgery, although this may be varied according to the patient's level of home care. The gingival tissues frequently shrink following surgery, especially interdentally, and instead of floss or tape the patient can be instructed in the use of an interdental brush.

Following periodontal surgery, the importance of regular maintenance cannot be overstressed, and the crucial role of the dental hygienist must be appreciated. Many studies have shown this aspect of treatment to be of more importance than the type of surgical procedure undertaken.

Application of fluoride for caries inhibition

The more obvious ways in which a clinician can reduce a patient's caries rate are by dietary advice and by improving oral hygiene. However, it is also of considerable benefit if topical fluoride treatment can be provided – a form of complementary therapy which is especially beneficial when the level of fluoride in the drinking water is low. Whatever the means of administration, two mechanisms can be hypothesized for the therapeutic effect of fluoride. The first is by substituting for hydroxyl ions in the hydroxyapatite crystal lattice of enamel. The fluorapatite formed is less soluble than hydroxyapatite, so rendering the enamel more resistant to decalcification by dental plaque products and also favouring recalcification when decalcification has occurred. The alternative way in which fluoride can work is by inhibiting the bacterial enzyme systems in plaque. Even very low concentrations of fluoride (2–10 ppm) will interfere with glucose metabolism by oral streptococci. The effect is more pronounced at pH 5.0, the level of acidity at which enamel is demineralized and caries can occur.

The simplest and most effective way of administering fluoride is systemically via the drinking water. Optimal therapeutic effect takes place at about 1.0 ppm. At lower levels the degree of caries reduction is less and at higher levels, up to 3.0 ppm, although the caries rate is reduced slightly further, unsightly, opaque, white spotting of enamel (enamel mottling) can result. At even higher levels the caries rate has been said to rise again, but this is more difficult to quantify due to the degree of enamel hypoplasia which occurs. When administered systemically, fluoride enters the extracellular fluid and from there is incorporated into the enamel either via the blood stream or indirectly from the saliva. Consequently, before the teeth erupt there is little the clinician can do apart from provide dietary advice on fluoride supplements. Once the teeth erupt, however, there is the opportunity for fluoride to be applied topically.

The proportion of fluorapatite in the superficial layers of enamel is increased by applying solutions of fluoride to the exposed tooth surface. An improvement in caries resistance may then result without the side effect of enamel mottling. Because immature enamel can take up more fluoride than mature enamel, this form of therapy is especially valuable in the period soon after tooth eruption.

In the past the ability of topical fluoride solutions to increase the proportion of fluorapatite in the surface enamel has encouraged the therapeutic application of strong (0.2–2.0% NaF) solutions of fluoride. Today it is less popular. Strong solutions of NaF can only be applied infrequently without running the risk of toxicity, and the regular, daily application of low concentrations of topical fluoride has a confirmed benefit. Higher concentration solutions are usually reserved for the patient at special risk or when some other complaint, e.g. dentine hypersensitivity, requires this form of therapy.

Fluoride toxicity

Apart from some vitamins, few therapeutic agents can be taken in excess without side effects developing. This is true of fluoride and care must be taken with topical agents because they contain high fluoride concentrations (Table 10.2). Following their use, accidental ingestion causes nausea and vomiting and has caused death. Any ingested dose greater than 1 mg/kg body weight must be looked on as being potentially toxic. Ingestion of

Table 10.2   Fluoride content of a range of topical fluoride preparations

Type	Available fluoride content
Toothpaste	0.1%
Mouthrinse	0.2% and 0.05%
Fluoride gel	1.2%
Fluoride varnish	2.4%

surplus fluoride (up to 5 mg/kg body weight) if detected early is best remedied by the immediate drinking of large quantities of milk. Unabsorbed fluoride ions are then converted to relatively insoluble, harmless, calcium fluoride. Ingestion of larger quantities warrants speedy hospitalization because fluoride is rapidly absorbed, with the side effects of excess salivation, nausea, vomiting and diarrhoea. The lethal dose is estimated to be about 14–15 mg/kg body weight. The risk of giving a fluoride overdose can be avoided by following a simple rule. Never apply topical fluoride so frequently and in such a concentration to a patient in the surgery for the total volume used to amount to a toxic dose, and never provide for home use so much rinse that it will amount to a toxic dose.

Fluoride therapy in the home

Systemic fluoride
Hygienists are fortunate in that they are less authoritative figures than dentists. Patients find it easier to communicate with them and hence they are more likely to be successful in an advisory role. In this way they can clear up misunderstandings and clarify for patients the link between the various systemically administered fluorides.

Fluoride can be introduced systemically in various forms namely as fluoridated salt, fluoridated milk, fluoride tablets and fluoridated drinking water. The ideal is via the drinking water but where this is lacking, fluoride tablets (1 mg fluoride in each tablet) are a useful alternative and can be incorporated in the food (therapeutic requirements: one tablet/day for children over 5 years, half a tablet/day for children under 5 years). Due to possible extremes in dietary preference, fluoridated salt and milk, although sometimes available, are too liable to variation in dose to be recommended for children.

Fluoride supplements are advised only if the drinking water contains less than the optimum fluoride level (1 ppm), and for this reason clinicians should be aware of the levels in the local water. Where a deficiency is known, supplementation of the diet with fluoride tablets can then be helpful, but the dose is reduced in accordance with fluoride levels in the local water. In cases of handicapping conditions, however, it may be advisable to increase the administered dose above the recommended level because the advantages of high caries resistance might outweigh possible aesthetic defects caused by mottling.

Fluoridated dentifrices

Almost all dentifrices (95%) on sale in the UK contain fluoride, either as sodium fluoride, sodium monofluorophosphate or a combination of both, usually at a concentration of about 0.1%. Sales of dentifrices and other oral hygiene aids have increased tremendously over the last decade or so, and it is probable that we have to thank the successful marketing expertise of the pharmaceutical manufacturers for much of the decrease in caries that has occurred over the same period of time.

Although there is a definite level at which systemic fluoride exerts its most beneficial effect, no such limit is placed on topical fluoride and it would appear that frequent applications of fluoridated toothpaste can only be beneficial. While this holds true for fluoride applied in the surgery and for cooperative adults using solutions at home, it is not always the case. When young children use fluoridated toothpaste without close supervision they tend to swallow a large proportion, and this in turn can possibly lead to unwanted systemic effects. It is therefore best to advise that children who live in fluoridated areas or are receiving adequate systemic fluoride therapy use an amount of toothpaste on their brush not larger than a small pea (0.3 g).

Fluoridated floss and wood points

These are normally used by adults and although they may be looked on as being of only marginal value, they are unique in that the fluoride they contain is placed precisely in the areas most at risk, namely the interproximal spaces. They are of further value in that an adult aware of the value of fluoride, and using the products for that reason, will also remove any plaque present in these regions.

Clinical materials and methods

Fluoride mouthrinses

Fluoride-containing mouthrinses are an invaluable means of caries inhibition. Two strengths are available, 0.2% and 0.05% sodium fluoride, the directions for both being that 10 ml is held in the mouth and swished around the teeth for 1 min before being spat out. Solutions for mouthrinsing are most effectively used under supervision in the surgery but can be provided for use by older children at home. To aid home use the manufacturers normally provide a cap for the bottle which, when filled, contains the required amount. Although the instructions appear unequivocal it is always best to give a demonstration in the surgery before providing solutions to take home.

While it would appear at first sight that use of the 0.2% solution would be more effective, its toxicity makes inadvisable its unsupervised use by children. Its use should be restricted to the surgery or, at most, only once a week at home under supervision. On the grounds of safety it is therefore best to recommend the use of 0.05% solution on a daily basis, a regime which has the advantage not only of greater safety but also of being more effective after daily use than the stronger solution at weekly intervals. For a worthwhile effect patients must use the solution for a year or more and avoid food, drink or rinsing with water for an hour afterwards. The best time for use is last thing at night.

Fluoride mouthrinses are of principal benefit to children, especially those who are suspected of being liable to caries or are undergoing orthodontic treatment. Nevertheless adults, too, can be helped, and fluoride mouthrinses can be prescribed to those who have difficulty in manipulating a toothbrush, who have an overdenture, or who might be susceptible to caries as a result of a deficiency in saliva flow, whether due to drugs, radiotherapy or other cause.

Topical fluoride solutions

Acidulated phosphate-buffered fluoride (APF) solutions (1.3% available fluoride) are still a popular chairside means of administering topical fluoride, but are more and more being reserved for cases of special need where regular daily use of 0.05% solutions are impossible or impracticable. The addition of sufficient acid to lower the pH to 2.8 ensures that more fluoride remains in the active form and that increased amounts of fluoride are absorbed by the enamel as a consequence of the slight surface decalcification caused during the process of application. Although unmodified APF solutions are available, the most popular have their viscosity artificially increased by the addition of sodium carboxymethyl cellulose, which converts them into more easily manipulable thixotropic gels. When using such materials only small quantities are needed, but careful control of moisture is essential otherwise contamination and dilution occur.

Although controversy exists as to whether plaque need be removed before application of topical fluoride, on dental health grounds it is difficult to justify leaving it in place. The quadrant or area is first isolated and the teeth cleaned and dried. A small amount of gel is transferred to the teeth with a swab, taking care to cover the entire surface and working the gel interproximally (Figure 10.7). After 60 s, surplus gel is aspirated off – never

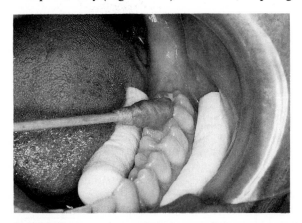

Figure 10.7   Application of fluoride gel to fissures and contact points of teeth by means of cotton swab

washed off – further teeth isolated and the process repeated. In this way minimum amounts of gel are used and the risk of toxicity reduced. Treatment should initially be repeated at weekly intervals for a month, preferably in the period soon after tooth eruption. Subsequently a single treatment can be given at yearly intervals at the time of the regular dental check.

Preformed disposable plastic trays are still obtainable by means of which, to save time, an entire arch can be treated with gel. After treatment for 60 s the tray is removed and excess gel expectorated. While saving time, such a method cannot be advised and must certainly be reserved for older children or adults. The danger of accidentally ingesting large amounts of gel is always present. There is also the possibility of absorbing large amounts of fluoride through the oral mucosa. For the same reasons the use of fluoride gel for caries prophylaxis of orthodontic patients undergoing fixed appliance therapy is contraindicated. The complex appliances tend to retain gel in the mouth and increase the dose of accidentally ingested fluoride.

Although principally reserved for children, caries prophylaxis for selected adults by means of fluoride gels is becoming increasingly common. It is particularly indicated for overdenture patients, when it can be applied in the surgery or can be given in small amounts for home application, a few drops being placed on the denture over the abutments once a week. Radiotherapy patients suffering from reduced salivary flow can benefit from a similar method of application; a close fitting, vacuum formed, soft acrylic splint is provided.

While the benefits of APF gels containing 1.2% fluoride are well established, a recently developed gel (Omnigel) contains stannous fluoride 0.4% and has been widely advertised. It is said to be suitable for surgery and home use and to suffer from neither of the disadvantages of the original stannous fluoride solutions, namely to cause tooth staining, or to have a short shelf life due to hydrolysis of the active ingredient. The benefits of this formulation, however, have not yet been fully established by clinical trial.

Fluoride varnishes
A very acceptable material for fluoride application is Duraphat, which contains sodium fluoride (2.3% available fluoride) in an alcoholic solution of natural varnishes. The material dries rapidly, is effective even if moisture control is not perfect, and is therefore especially suitable for young children. After achieving as dry conditions as possible, small amounts of Duraphat are applied to the pits, fissures and interproximal surfaces of teeth by means of either a small brush or a small piece of plastic foam (Figure 10.8). Once Duraphat was available for dispensation from a syringe fitted with a special wide needle. Very young or apprehensive children tended to be frightened by this method and the additional possible danger of accidental injection into the soft tissues led to its disuse.

Fluoridated prophylaxis paste
Fluoridated prophylaxis paste cannot be recommended as a routine method of applying topical fluoride. Whenever prophylaxis pastes containing the usual abrasive systems are used on teeth, small but significant amounts of enamel are abraded away (approximately 4 µm). If, to remove staining, the use of a prophylaxis paste becomes essential, then the deleterious effects of

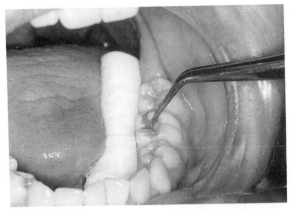

Figure 10.8   Application of Duraphat to fissures of posterior teeth by means of a pledget of cotton wool

the 'therapy' can be minimized if the prophylaxis paste used is one which contains fluoride. As a corollary, in the absence of stain, polishing of teeth should be performed with a rubber cup and a fluoridated dentifrice, never with prophylaxis paste.

Side effects of fluoride

In this health conscious age, few patients who are interested enough to be aware of the advantages of fluoride supplements will not be concerned to know of any side effects that have been recorded. The hygienist is well placed to reassure such patients and counteract worries caused by rumour. The commonest of these rumours is that fluoride, whether occurring naturally or by dietary supplementation, might cause damage to the fetus. Studies have shown that fluoride accumulates in the placenta but, reassuringly, the placenta also acts as a partial barrier against fluoride penetration to the fetus and so eliminates any potential danger of toxicity.

Other patients may be concerned whether fluoride is involved in the pathogenesis of cancer or Down's syndrome, and might quote statistics from papers published some 20 years ago. They may be reassured that such mendacious reports have been discredited by more recent, better designed investigations. No relationship can now be demonstrated between fluoride levels and the incidence of either of these two conditions.

Fissure sealants

Dental caries tends to occur in specific sites on the tooth surface. This was recognized at the turn of the century by G. V. Black who confirmed that the commonest sites for caries attack were the pits and fissures of molar and premolar teeth. In such sheltered sites plaque accumulates undisturbed and caries can follow in a susceptible individual. Later, it was only a small step to hypothesize that by excising and obturating the fissures in a tooth surface, so providing a smooth, easily cleaned and non-retentive surface, a patient's caries rate could be reduced. In due course the search for appropriate materials was accelerated by increased emphasis on preventive dentistry. This in turn led to modern fissure sealants being introduced to a public enjoying an improved standard of dental care and willing to accept the importance of sophisticated dental health measures.

Development

When the special liability of occlusal pits and fissures to caries was recognized, the practices of prophylactic odontotomy and extension for prevention became popular. These procedures were widely accepted by the dental profession despite involving the need to remove sound tooth tissue so that adequate access could be provided for insertion of the filling material. Later, when the acid-etch process was developed, there arose the opportunity for bonding suitable materials directly to enamel and obliterating fissures without the removal of tooth tissue. Due to its degree of polymerization shrinkage the natural first choice – poly(methyl methacrylate) – showed an unacceptable degree of microleakage at the resin/enamel junction. Only later when the bis-GMA resins were investigated did their reduced polymerization shrinkage make fissure sealants practicable.

The first fissure sealants to be introduced were unfilled resins and proved disappointing. Setting contraction still proved excessive and this, in association with their poor mechanical properties, often resulted in early loss of attachment. Even in successful cases it was difficult to assess the degree of sealant retention with certainty because the resins were transparent. Therefore, to improve the wear properties of the resin and reduce its polymerization shrinkage further, filler loading was introduced. Modern bis-GMA based fissure sealants now contain up to 50% filler loading, but their fluidity is sufficient to permit them to penetrate the fissure depths with ease.

The next development was the introduction of fissure sealants prepared from the so-called 'light cured' resins. Polymerization was initiated by light and allowed the operator to control the setting time more precisely. Simultaneously, to improve the visibility of resins without making their presence objectionable, white or coloured opacifiers were incorporated. The improvement in visibility allowed easy detection of defective sealant and permitted the retention rates and therapeutic effect to be accurately determined in clinical trials.

Finally, with the introduction of the glass ionomer cements a new type of sealant has been marketed which appears to have near ideal properties. It possesses minimal shrinkage, adheres to enamel merely by conditioning with polyacrylic acid, is not so sensitive to moisture contamination, and has the additional property of inhibiting caries by the release of incorporated fluoride.

Patient selection

Although a recent BDA/DHSS document has approved the use of fissure sealants as anti-caries agents, this is not to imply that fissure sealants can be used indiscriminately. Each case must be assessed individually because application of fissure sealants necessarily takes up valuable clinical time and the degree of cost effectiveness must vary in each case. The ideal time for their use is in the short period soon after eruption of the tooth, before the caries process has started. However, this might not be the most 'efficient' time. If fissure sealants were applied to each tooth soon after its eruption, numerous visits to the surgery would be involved which might be costly when expressed in terms of operator time occupied, parent time wasted and schooling lost. Often only in cases of special need such as handicapped patients or haemophiliacs, can this extra time and effort be justified on the grounds that tooth loss might give rise to exceptional management problems or be a health hazard.

Management problems can also occur when treating the normal, healthy patient. The first permanent molars erupt at about the age of 6 years, which is a time at which a proportion of children (usually those most in need) are intolerant of dental treatment. Soon after eruption the clinical crown is only partly exposed in the mouth, difficult to isolate from moisture by conventional means, and almost impossible to do so with rubber dam which would be the ideal method. Thus, although young children might be expected to gain maximum benefit, they are the group in which cooperation is sometimes a problem and the provision of effective fissure sealant therapy difficult. Finally, there is the anomaly that although the materials appear to be most useful in caries-prone individuals, they are the patients for whom treatment is most likely to result in disappointment. In a caries-prone child, even if fissure caries is inhibited, interproximal caries will soon follow (along, possibly, with loss of confidence in the operator's judgement) unless the application of fissure sealants can be guaranteed to be followed up with an effective regime of plaque control.

A practical method of patient selection is first to assess the caries rate by observation of the oral hygiene and the state, or absence, of the primary dentition. Where it is suspected that the caries incidence will be high, diet control and alternative preventive measures should at once be instituted before considering sealant therapy. When oral hygiene is good or it is suspected that good habits can be inculcated, fissure sealants can be provided for cooperative patients, preferably to the fissures of the first molars soon after all have erupted. If the upper and lower molars do not erupt almost simultaneously, and the need is urgent or the fissures deep and caries-prone, lower and upper molars may be treated separately on eruption. Subsequent visits can be timed to coincide with the eruption of the premolars (upper premolars tending to be more caries-prone) and second molars. A complete schedule of fissure sealing might then include molar and premolar fissures, buccal pits of lower molars and lingual pits of upper molars, and cingulum pits in incisors.

Table 10.3 Summary of clinical properties of some currently available fissure sealants

	Bis-GMA-based	*Glass ionomer-based*
Typical names	Delton, Helioseal	Fugi III
Matrix	Bis-GMA resin	Polyacrylic acid
Filler	Silica	Alumino-silicate glass
Cure	Chemical or light	Chemical
F·· available	No	Yes
Applications	All fissures	Wide fissures

Clinical materials and methods

Two types of fissure sealant are in common use (Table 10.3). The more popular and easier to apply is a filled (approximately 50% silica) bis-GMA resin, available in both self-curing and light-curing varieties. The other is a fluoride-releasing, glass ionomer cement which, while giving promise of great potential, is as yet not applicable to all cases and has a shorter history of clinical trial. The modes of application of the two materials differ slightly.

Resin-based sealants

Teeth to be treated are isolated and cleaned with pumice and water on a bristle brush. After washing off all traces of pumice, the etch solution or gel (30–50% phosphoric acid) is applied to the surface of the tooth on a small sponge, pledget of cotton wool or special brush, for a timed 30 s (Figure 10.9). The length of the etch period must be timed carefully and only modified in the case of primary teeth when, due to their slightly different anatomy and degree of calcification, the period of etch should be extended to 120 s.

To remove traces of plaque and food debris, the fissures can be dredged

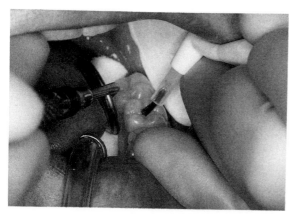

Figure 10.9 Etchant being applied to molar teeth with special brush prior to fissure sealing

with a fine probe for the first few seconds of etch. Instrumentation must be brief lest mechanical damage is done to the delicate etched enamel surface. Care must be taken to ensure that the entire surface likely to be covered later with fissure sealant is etched. If sealant is placed on unetched enamel the bond will be defective and allow leakage. After etching, the phosphoric acid is washed off for another 30 s and the enamel surface thoroughly dried. Between drying of the etched surface and application of fissure sealant the enamel must remain dry without the slightest contamination by water or saliva, otherwise bonding of resin to the enamel will not occur. In the event of accidental water contamination the surface must again be thoroughly dried. If saliva contamination occurs the surface must be thoroughly re-washed before drying.

If a self-curing resin is being used the components are mixed and allowed to run by capillary action into the fissures and over the surrounding enamel, transferring the resin with a sponge, pledget of cotton wool or an applicator provided by the manufacturers (Figure 10.10). Care has to be taken that the fissures are completely filled and air bubbles expelled. Once the resin has set the occlusion is checked, high spots identified with articulation paper, and reduced with fine diamonds. As a final measure a small amount of fluoride gel can be applied to the remaining etched surface to encourage recalcification.

When a light-curing resin is used the resin is transferred to the tooth with the same precautions as before, and the light directed onto the resin for 30 s from a distance of 1 mm or less. Care must be taken to avoid touching the unset resin with the light rod because removal of attached resin will be difficult, and if the tip is contaminated less light emerges on subsequent use. Concern once existed that polymerization of resin in the depths of the fissures might be incomplete with light-curing resins but more recent research has shown retention rates of sealant resins to be unaffected by the mode of cure.

Glass ionomer-based sealants

This type has the apparent advantage that the bond is less susceptible to moisture contamination, although the effect of saliva contamination is as

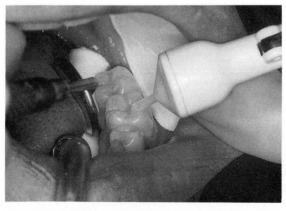

Figure 10.10   Fissure sealant being applied to teeth by means of disposable applicator

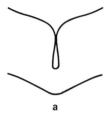 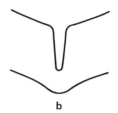

a   b

Figure 10.11   Diagram of fissure patterns suitable for two types of fissure sealant: (a) narrow fissures suitable for resin-based types; (b) broad fissure anatomy suitable for the more viscous glass ionomer cement type

adverse as for the resin-based variety. Because glass ionomer sealant is rather more viscous than resin sealant, it should be chosen only when the depths of the pits and fissures are patent and palpable with a probe (Figure 10.11). The clinical technique involves additional precautions to prevent dehydration of the cement which is susceptible to surface disintegration if allowed to dry out immediately after setting.

Following isolation and drying as before, but without cleaning with pumice, the enamel surface is conditioned with polyacrylic acid for 30 s, dredging the pits and fissures with a fine probe. After washing the conditioned surface and re-drying, the cement is mixed and beads of sealant transferred to the tooth with a probe, which is in turn used to help the cement fill the entire depths of the fissure. When sufficient material has been placed, the surface of the setting cement is protected with either 'cling film' or articulation wax. Once set the separating film is removed and excess cement quickly removed with a fine round bur. Finally a thin layer of light-curing resin is applied and cured, when final adjustments can then be made to the occlusal surface.

The future

Apart from the alternative use of providing a tough protective coating to a sealant restoration, resin-based fissure sealants may have a role to play even when penetration of the caries process to the dentine has occurred – provided that a perfect seal can be produced. Recent research has shown that under ideal conditions, and when applied over minimal caries, the metabolism of the remaining bacteria is inhibited and no further progression of the caries occurs.

Treatment of dentine hypersensitivity

Hypersensitivity of a tooth to hot or cold can result from caries, a leaking restoration or trauma, conditions known to be associated with pathological changes in the pulp. However, the commonest situation in which hypersensitivity arises is after gingival recession when toothbrush abrasion removes the overlying cementum or enamel, and dentine is exposed to the oral environment. In such cases the pain is produced by hot, cold, touch, and the application of citric and lactic acids. To date the phenomenon has always been shown to be associated with a normal pulp. While experience shows that the pain of dentine hypersensitivity usually diminishes with time, considerable relief can be obtained by prompt symptomatic treatment. Up until recently, treatment of the condition has had little in the way of a scientific basis. Not only were the mechanisms of pain production obscure, but clinical trials of potential therapeutic agents were made difficult by problems in measuring pain and the placebo effect of any form of treatment.

Dentine hypersensitivity is common, affecting about 15% of the population. The age range is wide, 20–70 years, with peak incidence in the 20–40 age group. Studies have shown it to be more common on the left side of the mouth (the side more easily cleaned by right-handed patients) where it is associated with lower plaque levels. The commonest sites to be affected are the buccal cervical margins of canines and first premolars. The presumption then is that gingival damage due to toothbrush abrasion causes recession of the gingivae which exposes root dentine, or even crown dentine if there is an element of enamel abrasion.

The mechanism for pain production is still obscure although most authorities agree that it is the result of fluid movement in dentinal tubules. Electron microscope studies have demonstrated that the non-sensitive surfaces of hypersensitive teeth or the equivalent areas of unaffected teeth show a much smaller number and much narrower tubules than sensitive areas. Fluid transport would therefore be expected to be much diminished.

A logical mechanism for the development of dentine hypersensitivity might then be as follows. After vigorous toothbrushing and minor trauma to the gingival margin, recession occurs with exposure of cementum. Because toothpastes contain abrasives, the cementum is rapidly worn away and the exposed dentine surface coated with a smear layer – an adherent coating produced by the action of mechanical cutting and abrasion – which has a protective action. The presence in the diet of organic acids, such as citric or lactic, removes the smear layer and exposes the patent dentinal tubules. Under favourable circumstances obturation of the tubules occurs with time, but in the interim noxious stimuli cause loss of surface fluid and pain due to fluid movement.

Diagnosis of dentine hypersensitivity is by exclusion, having eliminated all other possible causes of pain. Generally, affected teeth show very low plaque levels and the pain cannot be ascribed to the popular cycle of pain–neglect–plaque–pain so dear to advertisers of proprietary desensitizing agents. The pain is sharp and essentially short-term. If pain is prolonged then pulpal pathology should be suspected and the diagnosis changed. As a preliminary measure the sensitive teeth are rendered free of plaque and calculus, and dried – a procedure which may reveal further sensitive areas. Areas of hypersensitive dentine are best cleaned using a rubber cup and an abrasive-free fluoride-containing toothpaste such as Sensodyne F. If even this is intolerable, hypersensitive areas can be cleaned and dried with pledgets of cotton wool.

The first stage in treatment is prevention and an analysis of the diet is made to detect any causative factors. Drinks such as orange, grapefruit and apple juice are potent sources of citric acid and their use should be discouraged. Next, instructions must be given in toothbrushing and a technique taught which does not involve vigorous abrasion. Such simple remedies may be sufficient but if pain continues, active forms of treatment then start.

Fluoride mouthrinses are of great benefit to patients with dentine hypersensitivity and will also help to reduce the incidence of root caries. In such cases a rinse of 0.2% fluoride is used on a daily basis until the pain is relieved. To avoid any risk of toxicity, strict instructions should also be given to ensure that the mouthwash is never swallowed after use. The therapeutic effect of fluoride rinses is thought to be exerted by stabilizing the smear layer and preventing its removal. If unsuccessful with this simple measure, further treatment will then depend on whether the sensitivity is localized to one or two areas or is more generalized.

Localized hypersensitivity

This form is most effectively treated by means of Duraphat, a sodium fluoride-containing varnish. The technique requires the varnish to be applied to a clean, dry tooth surface by means of a small piece of foam plastic or cotton wool held in a pair of tissue forceps (Figure 10.12). To allow a prolonged action for the material, patients should avoid eating or drinking for a few hours. A further two or three applications at weekly intervals are usually sufficient, but in some cases more prolonged treatment is needed. With a cooperative patient, the layer of Duraphat can be maintained in place for 24 h or more by placing a periodontal pack around the treated teeth. The beneficial action of Duraphat is a consequence of the high level of fluoride (2.3%); it is unlikely that the vehicle can have other than a temporary obturating effect.

An alternative medication is Lukomsky's paste, which can be made up by a pharmacist, and contains equal parts (w/w) of glycerine, kaolin and sodium fluoride. It is rubbed into the exposed root dentine by a ball-ended burnisher

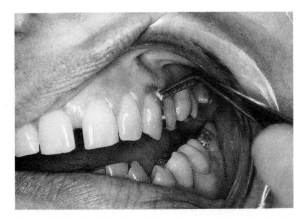

Figure 10.12   Application of Duraphat to sensitive dentine by means of pledget of cotton wool

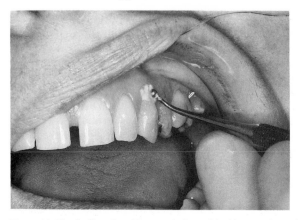

Figure 10.13   Sodium fluoride paste being rubbed into surface of sensitive dentine by means of ball-ended burnisher

or an orange wood stick, taking care to maintain isolation of the teeth (Figure 10.13). Like Duraphat, application must be repeated two or three times for maximum effect. Apart from any effect that the fluoride component might have, the act of burnishing should produce a smear layer or even increase its thickness.

When neither of the above measures produces a successful resolution of the pain, further treatment becomes necessary and involves placing an impervious layer over the sensitive areas. Dentine bonding agents are the first choice, for example Scotch Bond or Gluma although, to secure optimum adhesion with these agents, rubber dam is necessary and it is sometimes difficult to adapt the dam accurately to the margin of the tooth if gingival recession is a marked feature. An alternative form of treatment is therefore to apply a thin layer of a fluid glass ionomer cement, for example Ketac Cem. Glass ionomer cements have the further advantages that they are less affected by the presence of a small degree of moisture (but not saliva contamination) and the application of the appropriate conditioning agent – polyacrylic acid – is painless, especially if warm water is used for cleansing the conditioned surface. The final treatment, when all else fails, is removal of the pulp and root canal obturation.

Generalized hypersensitivity

Where hypersensitivity is mild but more generalized, one of the desensitizing toothpastes can be prescribed. A variety are marketed and Sensodyne and Macleans Sensitive have some therapeutic value. Apart from the action of the high level of fluoride which some contain, an additional mechanism by which they work can be inferred from electron microscope studies of teeth treated *in vitro*. With both of these toothpastes a layer of deposit derived from the incorporated abrasive is deposited on the surface, enhances the smear layer, and covers the patent tubule ends. In the case of Sensodyne the deposit is diatomaceous earth and in the case of Macleans Sensitive silica.

Alternative toothpastes contain similar abrasives but the effect is diminished because other ingredients such as citric acid or sodium lauryl sulphate are destructive of the smear layer.

When using a toothpaste it is obvious that unless the paste contacts the sensitive area there will be no beneficial effect. An adequate concentration in interproximal or other difficult to reach areas can be ensured by the use of paste-smeared Superfloss.

Polishing of restorations

The main reason for polishing permanent restorations is to give a smooth surface which not only retains less plaque but makes plaque removal easier. Well-condensed amalgam, properly cured composite and cast gold respond best to polishing and a high level of gloss can be produced (Figures 10.14 and 10.15). Not all restorations can be polished, however, and with cermets (metal particle reinforced glass ionomer cements) it is sufficient to achieve a smooth matt surface. A similar surface should also be achieved with glass ionomer cements if the glaze produced by setting in contact with the matrix band is lost.

Any polished surface is susceptible to corrosion and abrasion, especially in the mouth, and the appearance deteriorates. Subsequently the degree of long-term polish that can be maintained is determined by the patients's own level of oral hygiene. This should not deter efforts being made to achieve a high degree of polish because the initial appearance of a smooth, well polished restoration is pleasing to patients and they might be encouraged to maintain the appearance by greater efforts at oral hygiene.

Amalgam

A recently completed amalgam restoration has a matt grey appearance and will have been carved until it just maintains contact with the opposing and

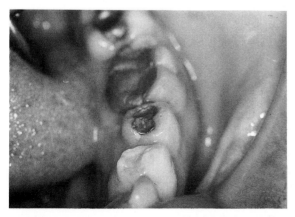

Figure 10.14 Old occlusal amalgam in lower left second premolar, showing rough surface and defective margins acting as plaque retention sites

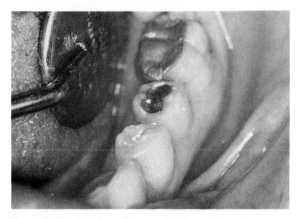

Figure 10.15   Amalgam illustrated in Figure 10.14 after polishing, showing smooth surface and undetectable margins

adjacent teeth. The polishing stage therefore involves first perfecting the shape of the surface anatomy, but with minimal removal of material, in order to maintain the important contact points. The entire surface is then polished, again with minimal loss of material.

Surface anatomy is perfected with a finishing bur. For occlusal surfaces a pear-shaped bur is ideal and with a light touch the amalgam is stroked from the central fissure area towards the enamel margin. When the amalgam is correctly contoured it is further smoothed with a rubber point, starting with a more abrasive and ending with a less abrasive type. A final polish is carried out when the amalgam has a uniform satin finish. Zinc oxide powder moistened with methylated spirits and used in a rubber cup or soft bristle brush is ideal, but for best results any contamination with saliva must be avoided. Finally, avoid overheating and pulp damage. This is especially liable to occur when using rubber points or cups at high speeds, and will be less likely to occur if the instrument tip is kept constantly on the move.

An interproximal surface is difficult to reach and cannot be highly polished. Flame shaped finishing burs are used to reach further into the interproximal region and approach the contact point. Linen strips coated with fine abrasive are then used between teeth but care has to be taken not to remove so much amalgam interproximally that the contact point is lost.

Occasionally it becomes necessary to remove interproximal ledges of amalgam when matrices have been poorly applied and amalgam has escaped through a cervical gap. Flame shaped finishing burs or abrasive metal strips are conventionally employed to reduce the overhang but such methods are very liable to cause damage to the soft tissues unless carefully used. An alternative which is more expensive is a special reciprocating handpiece used in conjunction with a triangular abrasive point. In many cases, when the advantages and disadvantages have been weighed, the best and most cost-effective way of treating an amalgam ledge is to replace the filling, taking care to ensure correct matrix placement.

Composite

A smooth surface results when a composite resin sets in contact with a matrix band. Every attempt should therefore be made by careful use of a matrix to ensure that the surface of an anterior composite requires no further finishing. When further finishing is required this is performed with abrasive discs, starting with the more abrasive and ending with the least abrasive. If required, a final lustre can be applied using a proprietary composite polishing paste containing micro-fine alumina as the polishing agent.

Posterior composites contain a higher proportion (up to 80% silica) of filler than anterior composites and are a little more difficult to polish. Fortunately the interproximal surface and contact point is formed by means of a matrix band and requires little attention. The occlusal surface is shaped first with either a tapered white stone or, more rapidly, with a fine composite-finishing diamond bur, and then with an alumina-impregnated rubber point. Final polishing is, as for anterior composites, with a proprietary composite polishing paste containing alumina.

Gold inlays and crowns

Cast metal restorations are polished before cementation and should not require further attention. At times, however, occlusal adjustment takes place after cementation and the rough surface has to be polished. Abrasive rubber points are the preferred instruments with progression from more to less abrasive as with amalgam. Every effort is made to avoid excess pressure and keep the point constantly on the move because, as with amalgam, the danger lies in overheating and subsequent pulpal damage.

Sharpening of instruments

With sharp hand instruments work is quicker and less painful. Tungsten carbide tipped hand instruments have a long working life and when blunt are either replaced or sent back to the maker for re-sharpening. Steel bladed instruments are less long-lasting but can be sharpened by the operator with minimal equipment. As a blade becomes blunt more force has to be applied to make it function and the risk of damage to the blade increases. When visible notching has occurred large amounts of metal must be removed from the blade to restore an intact edge, so running the risk of weakening the instrument. For this reason sharpening is performed at regular intervals before any blunting and chipping of the blade can be detected.

The method of sharpening is as follows. A flat Arkansas stone (silica) is cleaned and wetted with thin oil. Oil acts to prevent particles of metal impacting into the microscopic unevenness of the surface so destroying its abrasivity. For an instrument such as a push scaler with a single flat cutting edge, the cutting surface is placed flat against the stone which in turn rests on a flat surface (Figure 10.16). The instrument then remains still while the stone is moved smoothly backwards and forwards. A few strokes are sufficient to restore the cutting edge. Any swarf is removed by a light stroke on the flat surface.

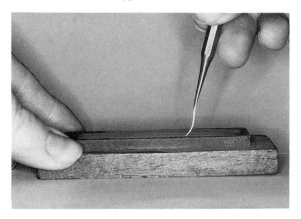

Figure 10.16   Method of sharpening instrument with a single flat cutting edge

Instruments with a curved pointed edge, such as the curved sickle scaler, require a different technique. The blade of the instrument is held in a pen grip against the stone with the flat upper face at an angle of approximately 110° to the surface of the stone (Figure 10.17). This time the stone remains stationary and the instrument is moved against the stone, maintaining the angulation of the upper face, with a combined stroke and roll so that a small section of the entire length of the blade is treated and a bright line produced. By repeating the procedure and slightly altering the angle of application, the entire cutting edge is brightened. Particular care has to be taken to ensure that the final third of the blade is sharpened. The procedure is then repeated on the opposite side. Any swarf on the upper face is removed with a small cylindrical Arkansas stone.

Instruments with a curved cutting edge such as curettes are sharpened using the same basic method as for those with a pointed edge except that the curved toe is left until the end. Once both sides have been sharpened, again using the pen grip, the toe is rounded in an analogous way. This section must be done separately, however, because considerable rotation has to be applied and great care must be taken if unwanted facets are not to be produced.

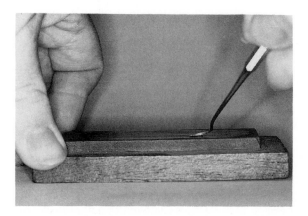

Figure 10.17   Method of sharpening instrument with curved cutting edge

Instruments can be rapidly sharpened with sandpaper discs mounted in a straight handpiece. This method is not normally advised because large amounts of metal are removed and the instrument quickly becomes useless. It is best to reserve it for sharpening damaged instruments only. Sharpening by conventional means, before the blade is blunted, is far preferable.

After sharpening, all instruments are cleaned with gauze, sterilized and stored ready for use. To ensure dry conditions which discourage corrosion and contamination by air-borne organisms, they are best left in a sealed autoclave bag.

Chapter 11

Special needs

For some categories of patient the long-term maintenance of their teeth requires special attention. With improved ways of preserving life and with increasing longevity of the population it is likely that greater numbers of patients will attend for treatment who have some degree of handicap or disability, whether developmental or acquired. Patients in these categories have special needs and considerable extra efforts are required of us if we are to satisfy those needs adequately. To simplify the approach to this aspect of dental care, modes of treatment for patients with the various types of special need will be described separately.

Motor disability

Motor disability may arise from a variety of causes. It may follow physical damage to the spinal cord or brain, e.g. paraplegia and cerebral palsy; be of developmental origin, e.g. spina bifida; or be the result of a disease such as Parkinson's, multiple sclerosis or myasthenia gravis. The significant problems of patients with a motor handicap are now better recognized and more attention is being paid to their solution. Problems may arise at various stages and are particularly acute when a wheelchair is the normal mode of transport.

Good access to the surgery is essential and ideally there should be easy access for a wheelchair. Steps are virtually impossible to negotiate single-handedly in a wheelchair or walking aid and the alternative of a shallow ramp should be provided. Corridors must be a metre wide and all doors at least 80 cm wide. Floor surfaces must be smooth without loose rugs or changes in level. When access is adequate for wheelchairs there will be no problems for less badly handicapped patients.

Once in the surgery a decision has to be made with wheelchair patients whether it is more convenient to treat the patient in the wheelchair or in the dental chair. Most patients can transfer to a dental chair if the wheelchair can be 'parked' alongside. The degree of help needed is best determined by patients themselves who are normally quite adroit at the necessary manoeuvres. Alternatively, experienced companions or relatives can be of great assistance. If transfer to the dental chair is difficult a detachable headrest may be attached to the back of the wheelchair and the wheelchair moved to a site convenient for the light and other equipment. When wheelchair patients are treated frequently in specialized units it may be best to use a special wheelchair lift which tilts the chair into the operating position.

During prolonged treatment provision must be made for any necessary 'physiotherapy'. Patients may need to exercise muscles to restore the blood circulation in order to avoid skin problems similar to bedsores. Handicapped patients can be questioned on this aspect beforehand and a rest from treatment taken at regular intervals. If oral hygiene instruction is to be given frequently to patients in wheelchairs, a sink at a suitably low level and lever handles on the taps are essential.

Plaque control methods will vary from normal only insofar as the patients lack normal control of their hands and fingers. In cases where manipulative skills are poor, the toothbrush can be adapted to give greater security of control. Elastic bands can be permanently attached to give extra support or the handle of the brush can be thickened with cycle handlebar grips or modified with cold-cure acrylic. Caries control by fluoride rinses is advisable. In severe cases chemical plaque control may be necessary although regular professional attention will be required to remove the resultant staining.

Mental disability

Many patients with a mild degree of mental disability (IQ 50–70) remain excellent dental patients. Although forgetful and in need of frequent reminders, they are enthusiastic and with understanding from the operator they come to relish a visit to the surgery. A patient with a greater degree of mental handicap than this finds oral hygiene difficult to perform and presents greater problems. Successful treatment then depends on a thoughtful and often prolonged approach. An added complication is that some forms of mental disability, e.g. Down's syndrome, can be associated with heart lesions and warrant antibiotic prophylaxis for some forms of treatment.

First, whatever the age of the patient, the support of the carer, whether nurse, parent or relative, must be recruited. Without their understanding of methods of achieving oral health and willingness to carry them out on a daily basis, little is possible apart from giving dietary advice and recommending topical fluoride application in the form of fluoridated toothpaste. With the help of the carer a full range of oral care is possible.

Next the confidence of the patient must be acquired, a process that can require several visits and involve slow, gradual introduction of the patient to the instruments and techniques of plaque and deposit removal. New items and actions are introduced by a process of show–tell–do and to ensure concentration and avoid discordant sensory stimuli the environment must be distraction-free without intrusive music. Repetition is an essential element of the introductory stage. Obviously threatening equipment must be inconspicuous, slow movements are performed and every attempt must be made to involve the patient in treatment by providing relevant, non-harmful items to take home, e.g. disposable dental mirror heads, oral hygiene leaflets and samples of toothpaste. The nature of the items can be selected according to the mental age of the patient and can be a useful form of home education for both patient and carer.

Finally, while successful progress to home therapy often occurs, oral health will have to be maintained by relatively simple methods. It is advisable to teach the scrub brushing technique and complex manoeuvres with floss silk and interspace brushes will be impossible. Chemical plaque control can be tried when all else fails. Chlorhexidine in the form of rinse or spray is very effective but the strong taste can produce a negative reaction. Cetyl pyridinium chloride and fluoride mouthrinse is a more acceptable but less effective alternative. It has to be acknowledged that extra time and effort must be made when treating patients with mental disability. There is no substitute for frequent maintenance and supervision, and constant reinforcement of the attitudes of patient and carer are essential.

The older patient

Elderly patients often suffer from a deterioration in oral hygiene leading to root caries and tooth loss unless efforts are made to bring the disease under control. Several factors contribute to the state of affairs. After retirement and loss of the daily routine that a career brings there is a tendency to eat irregularly, at short intervals, and not at the intervals dictated by work. Fermentable carbohydrate comes into contact with the teeth more frequently and caries follows. Retirement may also bring a reduction in income and cheaper foods are chosen with a greater proportion of refined carbohydrate. If this is also associated with loss of a spouse, an apathetic life style may be adopted and snack type foods chosen which require less preparation.

Apathy extends also to oral hygiene habits with plaque remaining in permanent contact with the teeth. Oral hygiene may be made worse if there is a lack of saliva. Hyposalivation is not inevitable with aging. Although some degeneration of salivary gland tissue takes place, the amount is not usually significant enough to cause functional difficulties. Hyposalivation is more usually a side effect of drug therapy, antidepressant drugs being a particular problem in this respect.

Oral hygiene in the elderly is maintained principally by the normal methods of adulthood, although an electric toothbrush can be useful if there is some degree of physical impairment. If there is recession of the gingivae, desensitizing treatment may be required and to avoid root caries a daily fluoride mouthrinse is to be recommended. If hyposalivation is causing a problem, an artificial saliva can be prescribed to aid lubrication of the mouth. A fluoride-containing aerosol spray type is best.

The difficulty that must be overcome is lack of enthusiasm. Elderly people are reputed to find learning difficult. This is an oversimplification. The elderly can learn complex tasks with great proficiency and are capable of intense intellectual effort. The problem lies in motivation. For the young person knowledge is of immediate benefit and the advantages of learning are apparent. For the middle-aged, too, learning is necessary to maintain their position in the world. The elderly, on the other hand, are no longer so pressurized and the techniques of improved oral hygiene and altered dental practices have to be reinforced by frequent repetition and clear identification of the advantages and goals to be achieved.

In the absence of cerebral pathology, much is possible. Once elderly people have been convinced of the need for good oral hygiene and have mastered the necessary techniques, they become model patients. Indeed, they often look forward to their review appointment and anticipate the social aspects with pleasure.

Endocardial disease and orthopaedic prostheses

A medical history which includes an episode of rheumatic fever must be viewed with suspicion. Rheumatic fever can be associated with endocardial disease and the bacteraemia caused by dental procedures such as extraction, scaling and root planing can result in an increased risk of a bacterial endocarditis, a condition which is frequently fatal even with treatment.

Opinions differ on the need for antibiotic cover for such patients during dental operations, some feeling that in the absence of a clinically detectable heart murmur antibiotic cover is unnecessary. Until the experts concur it is only sensible to provide antibiotic prophylaxis. For patients who are not allergic to penicillin the necessary regime is 3 g amoxycillin by mouth, under supervision, 1 h before the operation. Children under 10 years have half the adult dose and children under 5 have quarter the adult dose. Patients allergic to penicillin are given either 1.5 g erythromycin stearate by mouth 1–2 h before the operation followed by 500 mg by mouth 6 h later (with the same proportionate dose reductions for children as are appropriate for amoxycillin, but not exceeding 50 mg/kg body weight), or 600 mg oral clindamycin 1 h before the operation. For children under the age of 10 the dose of clindamycin is 6 mg/kg body weight. The same regime is required for patients with patent ductus arteriosus or septal defect. Prescription of the regime at intervals of shorter than 1 month is thought to be inadvisable in view of the possibility that resistant organisms may arise and, if present, will negate the beneficial effect of antibiotic prophylaxis.

When a special risk patient (one with a prosthetic valve, previous endocarditis, or a patient who has been prescribed penicillin more than once within the last month) is to be treated under general anaesthesia, the prophylaxis is slightly different. Those with no allergy to penicillin are given amoxycillin 1 g and gentamicin 120 mg, both intramuscularly, immediately before the operation and 500 mg oral amoxycillin 6 h later. With a patient allergic to penicillin the therapy changes to 1 g vancomycin intravenously over 60 min prior to the operation, followed by gentamicin 1.5 mg/kg body weight intravenously immediately before the operation.

The need for antibiotic prophylaxis for patients with a prosthetic hip or knee joint is more debatable. In this situation it is best to follow local practice and, when the surgeon responsible for the implant wishes to avoid any risk of infection, prophylaxis can be prescribed as for endocardial disease.

Immunocompromised patients

Patients with defects of their immune system are becoming increasingly common. Apart from developmental diseases such as hypogammaglobuli-naemia or agranulocytosis, a patient's immune response may be thera-peutically diminished following transplantation or treatment of neoplastic disease. In recent years HIV infection has become of significant importance.

Such patients are particularly at risk from infections acquired in the surgery and cross-infection procedures should be as those for hepatitis B. The patient is to be especially protected against the risk of infection from the operator, and organisms not normally pathogenic can be the source of severe infections.

Oral hygiene is very important. Patients in this category are liable to infections of the mouth. Oral candidosis, which gives rise to sore red areas, can be a particular problem. Chlorhexidine mouthrinses are a useful pro-phylactic measure, but when oral candidosis is present it is often the sign of a more generalized infection and treatment with systemic antifungal drugs is normal. Ketoconazole is the agent of choice at present but the risk of kidney damage must be borne in mind.

Diabetic patients

Diabetes is a common, incurable disease caused by reduction or lack of insulin production by the pancreas and characterized by high glucose levels in the blood. If occurring for the first time in a patient older than 40, it is often insidious in onset and the effects mild and controlled by weight reduction and modification of the diet. When diet modification is difficult oral hypoglycaemic drugs are helpful and help stimulate insulin production. In a young patient the disease is usually more sudden and severe, and there is a complete lack of insulin production. To maintain a near-normal blood glucose level rigid control of sugars in the diet is needed and injections of insulin are required.

The significance of diabetes to dentistry lies in the finding that insulin-dependent diabetics in particular appear to be more susceptible to periodon-tal diseases than normal and the periodontal state of some diabetics is characterized by rapid breakdown, a state which appears to be due to an altered host response. Research has shown that in insulin-dependent diabet-ics there is a defect in neutrophil polymorph function.

The goal to be achieved is a high standard of plaque control, and along with dietary control must go emphasis on oral hygiene if the teeth are to be preserved. At the same time it is important to eliminate other local irritants such as calculus or overhanging restorations. Generally those diabetics who find it easy to regulate their diet and maintain their blood glucose level also find it easy to accept the habits of regular oral hygiene. As a corollary, those who find difficulty in regulating their blood glucose require constant rein-forcement of the need for plaque control.

Diabetics also require consideration with regard to their appointments.

Normally they require three main meals each day with intermediate snacks. This means that the times they can attend the surgery may be restricted. Early and late times may coincide with meals, and mid-morning and mid-afternoon appointments may have to be avoided – or if necessary interrupted – to allow food intake.

Complex restorative dentistry

As the population becomes increasingly dentally sophisticated, so the demand for complex restorative procedures increases. Broken down teeth are replaced by crowns and the appearance of discoloured teeth improved by veneers. Weakened teeth can be reinforced by inlays, the mobility of loose teeth can be reduced by the use of interlocking crowns, and lost teeth can be replaced by bridges. Even after loss of all the teeth there is the possibility that dental function can be restored permanently by means of osseointegrated transmucosal implants.

Most forms of complex restorative dentistry merely involve precise replacement of the form of the missing tooth and, from the point of view of hygiene, normal methods of plaque control are adequate. Bridges and transmucosal implants require special attention because their shapes diverge from normal dental anatomy and their problems merit individual consideration.

Bridges

When applying oral health measures there are two kinds of bridge. Fixed and semi-fixed bridges are attached to the teeth on either side of the missing tooth or teeth and have pontics with relatively inaccessible fitting surfaces. Free-end cantilever or spring cantilever bridges are attached either to a tooth on one side of the missing tooth or teeth, or are attached to a tooth remote from the missing tooth or teeth. These latter types permit easy access to the fitting surface through one or both contact points.

In general there are few problems in ensuring good oral hygiene and the performance of dilatory patients can be encouraged by discussions of the costs involved if any of the complex restorations have to be replaced. Difficulties arise when the anatomical shape of the restoration is abnormal. Typically this is when the adjacent teeth are joined at the contact point. As mentioned above, this is always the case with fixed and semi-fixed bridges and only free-end cantilever and spring cantilever bridges allow the under-surface of the bridge to be cleaned via a contact point. Similar problems occur when united crowns are made or when interlocking inlays are prescribed.

Inaccessible fitting surfaces of bridges or the interproximal surfaces of united crowns necessitate the use of specially designed oral hygiene aids and the use of some form of floss threader must be taught. The simplest form of floss threader is a piece of thin, stiff plastic tape, one end of which is formed into a loop (Figure 11.1). By threading the floss onto the loop and passing the free end of the tape between the interproximal surfaces beneath the fused contact point, the floss is passed from the buccal to the lingual surface and after removal of the thread can be used in the normal way to clean the undersurface of the bridge or contact point. This technique is most easily performed on anterior teeth after a demonstration given with the patient observing by means of a mirror. The method works less well on posterior teeth where access is more difficult and the patient may have to supplement oral hygiene by use of an interproximal brush. An alternative to a floss threader is the use of Superfloss which has an integral threader – one end is stiffened to permit passage through the interproximal spaces. In extreme cases chemical plaque control by means of chlorhexidine mouthrinses may be the only way of maintaining plaque-free fitting and interproximal surfaces. Staining can then result and may need to be removed at regular intervals.

Osseointegrated implants

Restoration of a functional dentition for the edentulous patient by means of implants has been attempted for many years. Some success was achieved with subperiosteal metal frames but, in the long term, epithelial down-growth from the oral mucosa encapsulated the implant and rendered it liable to infection and sequestration. Predictable success was first achieved by Branemark using titanium implants placed within surgically created slots in the bone. After ensuring immobilization of the implanted structures, osseointegration occurs between bone and titanium via the molecule-thick layer of titanium oxide on the implant surface. On completion of osseointegration, superstructures are placed over the embedded sections and a complete denture – really an implant-supported bridge – inserted.

To ensure continued success of osseointegrated implants, the mainten-

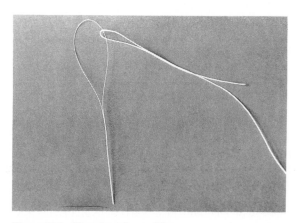

Figure 11.1   Floss threader and floss

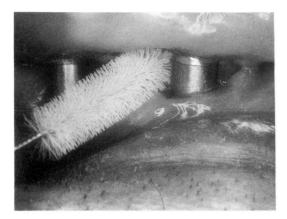

Figure 11.2 Osseointegrated dental implants. Spaces between abutments are being kept clean by means of an interdental brush

ance of plaque-free abutments is vital and the cleanliness of that part which pierces the mucosa has the highest priority. The spaces between the abutments are best kept clean with a 'bottle brush' type of interdental brush (Figure 11.2), and other abutment surfaces can be cleaned with Superfloss. Although careful daily use of these oral hygiene aids should keep the abutments plaque-free, review of all such patients by a hygienist is advisable at regular 6-monthly intervals. Any deposit can then be removed and oral hygiene reinforced. Hard deposits are removed with special polymeric-based instruments to avoid scratching or contaminating the relatively soft titanium surface by contact with another metal.

Removable dental prostheses

The patient with a removable dental prosthesis has special problems with oral hygiene. Although dentures are designed to be as hygienic as possible, inevitably the mouth of a patient without a prosthesis will be more healthy than one with. No matter what the design of the denture there is a biological price to pay. It is the duty of the clinician to keep the price to a minimum. Because the problems with the different types of prosthesis differ, those related to complete dentures, overdentures and partial dentures will be approached separately.

Complete dentures

The proportion of the adult population wearing complete dentures is becoming smaller as standards of oral hygiene improve and the incidence of caries diminishes. In the UK, nevertheless, 19% of adults wear complete dentures and their specialized needs are all too infrequently recognized. Plaque can accumulate on dentures as it can on teeth, and the consequences are staining, calculus formation and bacterial infection. The role of the hygienist is to institute a denture cleansing routine which is effective and acceptable to the patient. The majority of complete denture wearers are elderly and, following the insertion of new complete dentures, efforts have to be made to overcome by enthusiasm and practical help the problems of learning and decreased manual dexterity so often present in this section of the population.

Denture hygiene instruction should begin before replacement dentures are fitted by the demonstration of plaque on previous dentures. Disclosing solution is highly effective, and emphasizes the need for a proper denture cleansing routine (Figure 11.3). For immediate dentures instruction is given at a review stage. Although instructions on the cleansing of dentures will have been given when the dentures were inserted, it is sensible to review procedures and reinforce motivation.

The simplest method of cleansing dentures is with soap and a soft nail-brush or with denture toothpaste and a special denture brush. While having the advantage of cheapness and simplicity, the methods have drawbacks. The denture becomes slippery and the patient must be warned to clean the dentures over a towel or basin of water, either of which will break the fall and prevent fracture if the denture is dropped. The other draw-back is that patients' manual dexterity may be diminished and cleaning may be inefficient even when a large, specially designed toothbrush is bought.

An alternative is to use an immersion cleanser. Immersion cleansers come in tablet form and are added to warm water to form a solution in which the denture is immersed for a specific period of time. The most effective immersion cleansers contain detergents or hypochlorite either alone or in combination and a few contain hydrochloric acid. The action may be aided by bleaches (peroxides and borates) and proteolytic enzymes. While hypochlorite is a very effective plaque-removing agent and hydrochloric acid will remove calculus, both cause corrosion of metals and must never be used when the denture has a metal base. Patients should also be warned to follow carefully the instructions for use. Hot water will cause stress relief and distortion of acrylic dentures, and if bleaches are also present whitening of the surface resin occurs.

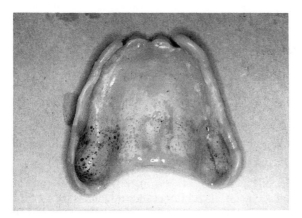

Figure 11.3 Plaque on distal half of complete upper denture revealed by disclosing solution

Partial dentures

On functional grounds, partial dentures may be divided into two extreme types: those supported by the natural teeth and those supported by the soft tissues and bone. An intermediate group also exists in which support is divided between teeth and bone. Dentures with tooth support must be designed to meet much greater stresses, comparable in magnitude to those resisted by the natural teeth. For this reason they have a metal base, usually cast cobalt/chromium alloy. Those with only soft tissue support usually have an acrylic resin base. Nevertheless, patients often prefer the feel of a thin metal base and for this reason a metal base may be needed. It may also be prescribed if stresses are unusually high, e.g. when the lower incisors contact an upper base due to a complete overbite, or when a prominent palatal torus produces a point of weakness or stress concentration.

The majority of partial dentures depend for their efficient functioning on an integration with the remaining teeth. Resistance to masticatory forces is provided by occlusal rests which fit into slots in either teeth or restorations. Resistance to vertically displacing forces is provided by direct retainers or clasps which fit into undercuts on the axial surfaces of the crowns of teeth (Figure 11.4). Resistance to lateral displacing forces is countered by contact of the denture base with non-undercut tooth surfaces. In partial dentures of an advanced design, resistance to various forms of displacing force is provided by the base entering machined channels in crowns or by spring loaded devices entering natural or artificially created undercuts.

The prevention of any further caries must be a high priority. If caries of a tooth contacting a partial denture occurs, restoration is difficult if the original tooth/base contact is to be re-established. If caries of an abutment

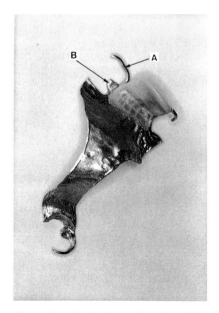

Figure 11.4   Typical metal-based partial denture. Arrows point to: clasps (A) and rests (B)

tooth occurs, the denture must very often be replaced. Even greater problems occur if a tooth is lost. Loss of an abutment tooth means that the denture must be replaced, but because many partial dentures depend for their continuing satisfactory support on maintenance of the remaining teeth as parts of an intact arch, unless the denture is of a simple, acrylic-resin base soft tissue supported type, loss of any tooth often means that the denture must be replaced. This may be very inconvenient, because following tooth loss a temporary denture will be required until the initial rapid resorption phase of alveolar bone is over.

The patient with a partial denture needs the help of a hygienist because there will be serious financial consequences if further caries occurs. Instruction in the cleansing of the denture, on the lines described above for complete dentures, is secondary to ensuring that oral hygiene is of a very high standard. Patients must be told not to leave the denture in their mouth when carrying out procedures. When examining the mouth hygienists should also include examination of the partial denture. Special note should be made of any wear of either the denture or abutment teeth, or of loss of retention.

Overdentures

Overdentures are provided primarily when there is fear that if teeth are lost the resulting alveolar bone resorption will compromise denture stability. Consequently, selected tooth roots are preserved after removal of their crowns and the retained root preserves alveolar bone which in turn provides lateral stability for the denture (Figure 11.5). The exposed root surfaces also serve to provide extra vertical support to the denture; hence, overdenture therapy may also be advisable in cases where the face height is to be increased and extra stresses will be imposed on the denture-bearing area.

Inevitably, if root surfaces are to be covered by a denture base there will be the risk of further caries; regular attention by a hygienist will help

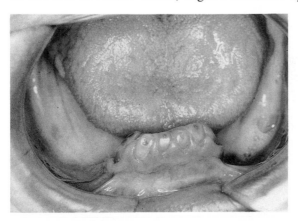

Figure 11.5 Retained roots acting as overdenture abutments and retaining alveolar bone in the mandibular anterior region

preserve roots which would otherwise be quickly lost, and patients must be warned to brush root surfaces as well as teeth. Extra precautions include prescription of fluoride mouthrinses (0.05% daily) or use of APF (acid-ulated phosphate-buffered fluoride) gel (1 drop weekly applied to the fitting surface of the denture over the root surfaces). Alternatively, after brushing the teeth, the patient can apply a small amount of fluoridated toothpaste to the fitting surface of the denture over the root face to prolong the period of fluoride treatment.

Denture stomatitis

Denture stomatitis is usually found beneath complete upper dentures but can occur beneath any form of oral prosthesis, including orthodontic appliances. Alternative names for the disease are denture-associated candidosis and denture-sore mouth. It is characterized by redness of the denture-bearing area and comes in three forms. Type I, the least severe, shows discrete areas of redness beneath the denture. In type II the redness covers the entire denture-bearing area, and in type III the redness is associated also with papillary hyperplasia (Figure 11.6). The cause is proliferation of a fungus (normally *Candida albicans*) in the plaque deposited on the denture and the predilection for an upper denture may be a consequence of its relatively good retention and the consequent fluid stasis beneath it. Its incidence is greatest in the elderly and it has been claimed to occur at some time in one-third of the denture-wearing population. While the symptoms are relatively mild the condition tends to occur in individuals susceptible to infection and, apart from the local elimination of disease, treatment is provided to prevent spread to other sites.

Diagnosis is made on clinical grounds and confirmed by swabbing the fitting surface of the upper denture and identifying large amounts of candida in the plaque. When, in type I cases, only small amounts of candida are isolated, the cause of the redness may be ascribed to trauma and the source of trauma – usually an ill-fitting denture – either removed or corrected.

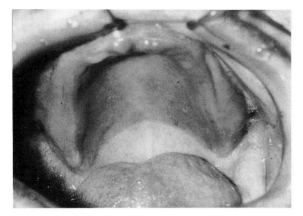

Figure 11.6   A typical case of type III denture stomatitis in which there is inflammation and papillary hyperplasia of the maxillary denture-bearing surface

Except when trauma is diagnosed, treatment involves improvement of oral hygiene and disclosing solutions are helpful for identifying plaque both in the surgery and at home. The aim of preliminary treatment is a permanent improvement in oral hygiene and methods of cleansing dentures have to be emphasized. If removal of plaque by mechanical means is difficult, immersion in hypochlorite solutions is usually effective. When no improvement can be made by these methods, locally applied antifungals are prescribed. Nystatin pastilles are excellent but have a strong taste which patients object to and a more acceptable choice is miconazole oral gel, a few cm of which are squeezed from a tube onto the fitting surface of the denture after each meal. Treatment is carried on for about 6 weeks to ensure that all spores are killed, but relapse is common unless the conditions predisposing to the infection are eliminated.

Some resistant cases are associated with a systemic defect, either anaemia, diabetes or immunocompromising condition. For this reason particularly florid or resistant forms should be regarded with suspicion and the appropriate tests prescribed.

A condition which is frequently associated with denture stomatitis is angular cheilitis where the angles of the mouth are red, cracked and painful (Figure 11.7). The condition is rationalized as being initially due to a reduction of the height of the lower third of the face due to excessively worn dentures or dentures in which the upper anterior teeth give inadequate lip support. In either case the skin at the corner of the mouth becomes creased and macerated by escaping saliva. Infection from an associated denture stomatitis can then follow.

Treatment involves correction of any denture fault and treatment of the infection after identification of the offending organism. Swabs of the angles of the mouth and the anterior nares (a likely site for cross contamination) are taken. *Candida albicans* and/or staphylococci are the usual organisms found. Fusidic acid ointment will eliminate staphylococci and miconazole ointment is effective against both *Candida albicans* and staphylococci.

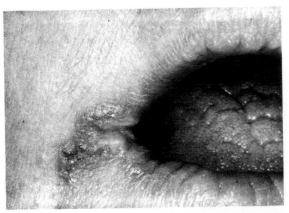

Figure 11.7   A typical case of angular cheilitis. *Candida albicans* was isolated from the area

Chapter 12

The dental team

Integrated treatment

To ensure the most efficient treatment of patients, especially those suffering from various forms of periodontal diseases, it is essential that each member of the dental team knows their area of responsibility and is able to relate it to those of the other members of the team. Previous chapters have outlined the overall management techniques, but this section attempts to describe those points that are specific to each clinical team member.

Dentist

The dentist has the ultimate responsibility for management of the patient, including legal accountability for the correctness of the actions of the other team members.

Responsibility starts with the process of screening and detection of disease, followed by a thorough assessment. Making a diagnosis precedes discussion of appropriate treatment options with the patient. For the patient with chronic inflammatory periodontal disease, referral to a dental health educator or a dental hygienist should be considered.

Before referral it is important that the patient is fully aware of their problems, the treatment objectives and the procedures to be undertaken by the health educator or hygienist. It should not be left to the ancillary to explain to the patient the reason for his/her attendance.

It is also the responsibility of the dentist to monitor the progress of the patient and following initial therapy to recheck the periodontal state and advise on further therapy.

Dental assistant

The tasks of the dental assistant are not only to assist the dentist at the chairside and act as a witness to what is said, but also to serve as a dental health educator. The patient will often, in the absence of the dentist, take the opportunity to ask questions about the treatment. It is important, therefore, that the assistant understands the general treatment principles and is able to relate these to the patient under care.

Dental hygienist

Hygienists are the main link in the management of the periodontal patient. They must be able to work with the information provided by the dentist, and produce specific plans that can be applied to the patient under care.

To discuss the problem and the necessary action, the hygienist must be a good communicator with a pleasant and persuasive personality. An open and honest approach is necessary, and it is essential that hygienists have experience of all the techniques and methods that they advocate.

In addition to communication skills, the hygienist is called upon to undertake very demanding clinical procedures, which must be carried out in a manner that retains the sympathy and confidence of the patient. Close liaison with the referring dentist is essential with both having a common approach on appropriate oral hygiene methods, so that conflicting advice is not given to the patient. It will be necessary for the hygienist to judge when to refer the patient back to the dentist, and for the average patient who might require initial therapy taking perhaps three or more visits, this would be an interval of approximately 3 months.

Receptionist

The receptionist acts as the public relations face of the practice. The attitude of the patient will often be tempered by the way in which they have been handled by the receptionist. A sympathetic, helpful approach is essential with patients who are attending the practice.

Periodontal screening, assessment and monitoring

One of the more important procedures that the general dental practitioner can undertake is to screen patients attending the practice for signs of inflammatory periodontal diseases. Recently the Community Periodontal Index of Treatment Needs (CPITN) has been developed as a screening tool, most notably by the British Society of Periodontology. The version of the index used is detailed in the Appendix. As the CPITN is a poor treatment needs indicator, and is rarely used by community services, it has recently been suggested that the term 'Basic Periodontal Examination (BPE)' be used in its place.

The Basic Periodontal Examination needs to be supplemented by appropriate radiographs. For the patient without any signs of overt disease, bitewing radiographs or an orthopantomograph will give information on the posterior bony contour, and these should be complemented by periapical views of the anterior teeth, preferably taken by the long-cone parallel technique.

For a full periodontal assessment or monitoring, more detailed indices than those used for screening are required. These should include the following assessments:

1. Gingival health using a bleeding or gingival index.
2. Probing depths.
3. Mobility using a mobility index.
4. Plaque deposits using a plaque index.

Information concerning periodontal probing is given below. Details of the other assessments may be found in the Appendix.

Periodontal probing

Despite arguments as to the significance of periodontal probing depths in the progression of periodontitis, they do give an accurate picture of the progress of disease and are one of the most important prognosticators, together with mobility, of the likely life of the tooth. Such an important criterion deserves consideration.

Probing depth varies according to the following factors:

1. Type of probe.
2. Probing force used.
3. Depth of the pocket.
4. Amount of inflammation in the area.
5. Access to the pocket.
6. Presence of features which impede the probe such as calculus, the presence of restorations, or root surface features such as furcations.

The type of probe, especially the diameter of the tip, will determine the force that is applied to the tissues and thus the degree of penetration of the junctional epithelium. The World Health Organization (WHO) recommends a tip diameter of 0.5 mm. A number of probes have been designed to meet this specification and three will be described, namely the Williams probe, the WHO probe and the University of North Carolina probe (Figure 12.1), although many other manufacturers are in the process of changing their probe tip diameters.

The Williams probe has irregular markings at 1, 2, 3, 5, 7, 8, 9, and 10 mm depths. These irregular gaps help in assessing the depth of the pocket and have been shown to be less confusing than probes with regular markings. The modified WHO probe has a 0.5 mm ball end and instead of millimetre graduations has two bands from 3.5 to 5.5 mm and from 8.5 to 11.5 mm. This enables not only a Community Periodontal Index of Treatment Needs coding (CPITN) to be assessed but also allows probing depths to be

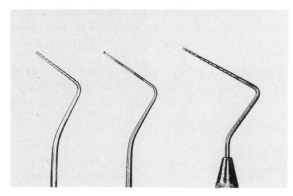

Figure 12.1 Suitable probes for periodontal probing depth assessment. From left to right: the Williams, World Health Organization and University of North Carolina periodontal probes

measured. The University of North Carolina probe has 1 mm markings, but every fifth millimetre band is characterized in black, so that the pocket depth is easily checked.

The probing force used determines the penetration of the probe into the junctional epithelium. The latest recommendations are that a very light force should be used, of the order of 15–25 g. This is a force which, if applied to a periodontal probe placed under the fingernail, would not cause any discomfort. To enable the force to be controlled, constant force probes have been developed (Figure 12.2) which prevent the application of excessive force to the base of the pocket.

The depth of the pocket and the amount of inflammation present will also determine the probing depth reached. The greater the degree of inflammation in a pocket, the further the probe penetrates into the junctional epithelium. For this reason the probing depths should always be reassessed after initial therapy has reduced inflammation.

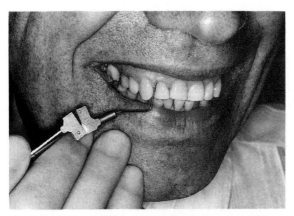

Figure 12.2 A constant force probe in use. The spring in the handle can be set to limit the force applied to the probing tip

The access to the pocket and the presence of root surface deposits will determine the ease with which the pocket can be entered by the probe. The classic example is furcation pocketing where, because of the morphology of the root, the full extent of the lesion cannot be explored. This should be borne in mind when examining periodontal pockets.

Probing sites

Probing depths may be measured at two, four or six sites around the tooth (Figure 12.3). The more sites assessed the more accurate the information gained and the fewer the periodontal lesions that will be missed. At the simplest level, measuring mesial and distal sites on each tooth will identify the great majority of problems, as it is unlikely that a tooth with, for example, a mid-facial lesion, will not also have a mesial or distal lesion. A more accurate method is to measure the mesial, distal, facial and lingual pockets. The most accurate method of all is to measure the probing depths on the mesial, distal and mid-facial or lingual on each side of the tooth, giving six readings per tooth.

Recording information

Many different systems are available for recording the information obtained from probing. The system described in the Appendix allows the information to be recorded sequentially over a period of time. This permits both the operator and patient to assess the progress of the condition.

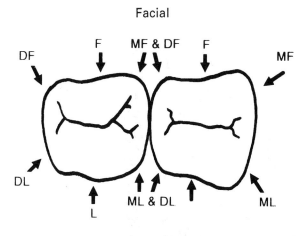

Figure 12.3 Sites at which probing depths may be measured

Use and interpretation of radiographs

Prior to discussing the use of radiographs it is important to consider the hazards of dental radiography and put these into perspective in everyday life. We are surrounded by naturally occurring background radiation. This background radiation is of two types, terrestrial radiation and cosmic radiation.

Terrestrial radiation is emitted from naturally occurring radioactive substances found in the ground. Examples of these include uranium and thorium present in various rock formations. With the passage of time, these substances undergo radioactive decay and lose their radioactivity, some of which is given off in the form of radon gas. Cosmic radiation comes from sources elsewhere in the universe. This radiation is of high energy and originates from stellar explosions deep in space, with a less powerful type of cosmic radiation coming from solar flares on the surface of the sun. Much of this type of radiation is filtered by the earth's atmosphere, particularly in the ozone layer.

Exposure to radiation has two basic effects on the body which are referred to as somatic and genetic. The somatic effect is seen in the individual exposed to radiation and this may be of the acute variety which may appear within days or weeks, or may be long-term, sometimes not appearing until many years after exposure. The genetic effects are seen in the offspring of the person exposed.

It is important to note that radiation exposure has a cumulative effect on the body and each exposure adds to the total, therefore diagnostic radiographic procedures must be kept as low in number as possible. For the purposes of dose limitation the population is divided into three groups:

1. Those receiving diagnostic or therapeutic radiation (patients).
2. Those who are occupationally exposed (such as radiographers).
3. The public at large.

Minimizing the ill effects from dental radiology

1. The single most important way to reduce patient dosage is only to take a radiograph when there is a specific clinical indication. If the information that a radiograph will reveal will not particularly help in the management of the case then it should not be taken.
2. The X-ray set should be in optimal condition and have been regularly serviced and should possess an accurate timer.
3. The operator should be properly trained in the taking of radiographs.
4. A fast film should be used.
5. Correct film processing is essential using developer and fixer solutions which are optimally active. If these solutions are ineffective then the diagnostic quality of the developed film will be limited.
6. The clinician should be shielded when the X-ray equipment is in use and should never hold the film in the mouth during exposure.
7. Ensure that no other person is unnecessarily exposed to radiation during the taking of a dental radiograph.
8. Patients should be protected by a lead apron.

9. The clinician should wear a film badge for a period of time to assess the levels of radiation to which he is exposed. Wearing a badge for 1 month every year would be sufficient.

The recently accepted acronym to remember when taking dental radiographs is ALARA; these letters stand for As Low As Reasonably Achievable and indicate the need to keep medical and dental radiography to a minimum as proposed by the International Commission on Radiological Protection.

Intraoral radiography

The intraoral films that are undoubtedly of most use to the dental surgeon or auxiliary are bitewing and periapical radiographs. These films reveal in good detail any abnormalities of teeth and their supporting structures. A bitewing film will reveal the presence of approximal caries, or recurrent caries under a restoration as well as the presence of calculus deposits and the degree of bone involvement in early inflammatory periodontal diseases. A periapical film will reveal more information but over a smaller area as only a few teeth can be viewed on a single radiograph. The periapical film reveals the whole structure of the crown and root and any disease or abnormality associated with it. For example, if a tooth has an abscess and it is not certain whether it is of pulpal or periodontal origin, a periapical film would be the one to take.

Bitewing radiographs

These are the easiest intraoral films to take. Positioning involves the patient biting on a tab, holding the film, which is placed between the opposing molar and premolar teeth. The cone of the X-ray set is then aligned so that the central ray will hit the film at a 90° angle, as shown in Figure 12.4. If this

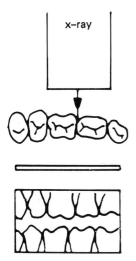

Figure 12.4   Suitable positioning of the X-ray apparatus to allow the central beam to be at right angles to the bitewing film

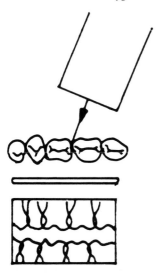

Figure 12.5   Incorrect positioning results in a film showing overlapping contact areas

angulation is incorrect then the contact points of teeth can overlap which may mask the presence of approximal enamel caries (Figure 12.5). Films can be purchased with the paper biting tab already in place, or self-adhesive tabs can be purchased which can be fixed to the film in the surgery. When positioning the film in the mouth the anterior edge should lie just distal to the canine.

Periapical radiographs
These are more difficult to take than bitewings because the cone of the X-ray set needs to be carefully positioned with respect to the film. Incorrect positioning will result in distortion of the image or even totally missing the tooth under investigation. There are two techniques which can be used. One approach, the bisecting angle technique, involves placing the film in the mouth and then positioning the X-ray set to throw an image on to the film which will produce minimal distortion of the tooth. This type of radiograph is normally used for dental X-ray sets with 'short' cones which allow the target (X-ray source) to skin distance to be about 20 cm. A diagrammatic representation of the bisecting angle technique is shown in Figure 12.6. The second method of periapical radiography is known as the paralleling technique or 'long cone' technique.

This gives a more accurate image of the tooth on the film because the film is held in a position which removes the element of compromise used in the bisecting angle method. The film is held in a special film holder which allows it to be placed parallel to the tooth and then the X-ray set cone is carefully attached to the holder, so that the resulting image is not subject to distortion. This is demonstrated in Figure 12.7. The disadvantages of this method are that it is more time consuming and also some patients cannot tolerate the film holders. In experienced hands the technique allows accurate images to be taken.

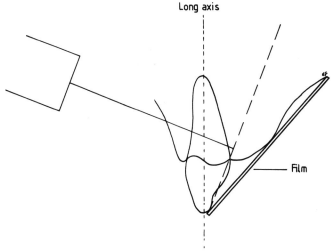

Figure 12.6 The X-ray set positioned so that the central beam is at 90° to a line which bisects the angle formed between the long axis of the tooth and the position of the film. In practice radiography books recommend an average angle for the beam angle

Extraoral radiography

The most useful radiograph which allows a general examination of the maxillary and mandibular teeth together with the surrounding structures is the dental panoramic tomogram. This is more usually referred to as an orthopantomogram (OPT/OPG). These films are of great value because not only will they show the presence of cysts, fractures, buried or impacted teeth, but they will also give a general indication of alveolar bone loss in periodontal disease. Because a degree of distortion is present in all of these films it is not advisable to use them as a means of identifying approximal

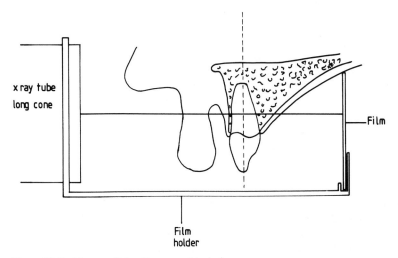

Figure 12.7 The parallel or 'long cone' technique

caries. The radiation dosage that a patient receives from an OPG is about the same as that for six periapical films. Figure 12.8 shows an example of an OPG in a patient with advanced inflammatory periodontal disease.

Processing of the film

The processing of a film begins with developing the image produced by the X-rays on the film emulsion, which itself consists of silver bromide crystals in a gelatin base. The developer solution is a reducing agent which induces the formation of a latent image on the film, by altering the crystal structure of the silver bromide so causing the deposition of small amounts of silver. The time taken to develop a film should be between 3–4 minutes at 20°C. The film is then removed from the developer, washed in water and placed in the fixer solution.

Fixer is a solvent for unexposed silver bromide which it removes from the film to produce the clear radiograph which can be viewed after it has been washed and dried. The time needed to fix a film is twice the time needed for it to 'clear', in other words when a sharp image is produced. The effectiveness of fixer is not temperature-dependent and the solution will remain effective for considerably longer than developer. This process is now quite commonly undertaken by automatic film processors which will carry out all the stages and provide a fully developed film which is ready for viewing.

Film faults

There are three basic reasons why unsatisfactory radiographs are produced. These include poor clinical technique, incorrect exposure time and faulty processing. If clinical technique is poor this is usually due to incorrect film positioning in the mouth, or angulation of the X-ray set.

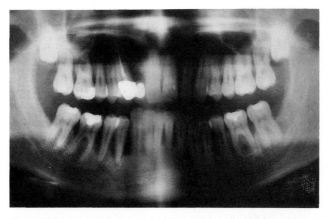

Figure 12.8   An orthopantomographic radiograph showing advanced bone loss due to periodontitis. The bone loss in the incisal region is difficult to see due to the superimposition of the spinal shadow

Excessive bending of the film before placement in the mouth, exposing the film back to front and not having the X-ray beam correctly aimed are all quite common. An incorrect exposure is usually due to setting the wrong time on the exposure dial. Processing faults are usually due to incorrect temperature of developer or using solutions which are exhausted.

Interpretation of dental radiographs

The radiographs which will be most used in clinical dental practice are the OPG, bitewings and periapicals, and therefore being able to interpret these films is important. The OPG provides gross information on the mineralized structures related to the mouth. It will reveal the presence of jaw pathology such as cysts, neoplasms and unerupted teeth. It will also reveal gross caries and give the clinician an idea as to the amount of bone loss which has occurred in periodontal diseases.

However, as in all techniques the OPG has limitations, some of which include poor clarity in the incisor region, marked distortion if the patient's head is not positioned correctly in the machine, and the possibility of a secondary image developing which may mimic pathology.

Intraoral films reveal in good detail what is happening to teeth and their supporting structures. Periapical films demonstrate the whole tooth from crown to apex and show the presence of caries, endodontic irregularities, periapical pathology as well as the extent of alveolar bone loss in periodontal disease. The periodontal ligament space can also be evaluated, and if this shows widening, pathology may be present. The lamina dura is the white line

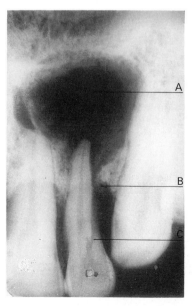

Figure 12.9 A periapical film showing a large dental cyst (A), marked bone loss due to periodontitis (B) and a lateral invagination in the root (C)

seen lining the bone of the tooth socket next to the periodontal ligament space. If this is not seen as a continuous line around the periodontal ligament space then some abnormality is present which requires further investigation. The interpretation of a periapical film taken using the paralleling technique is shown in Figure 12.9.

Bitewings have an advantage over periapicals by showing teeth in both maxillary and mandibular arches but they will not reveal the periapical area. They are indicated to check for caries, early periodontal disease and over-hangs on posterior teeth. They will generally show the coronal third of the root of upper and lower teeth. The evaluation of a bitewing is shown in Figure 12.10.

The techniques of dental radiography are many and varied and their interpretation can at times be confusing. It should be noted that radiographs are an adjunct to clinical diagnosis and should not be considered as a substitute for it.

Ethical dental hygiene practice

Despite recent government moves to reduce the legal privileges of pro-fessional bodies in the UK, the obligation remains for members of pro-fessional bodies to maintain high ethical standards. The ethical obligations incurred by members of a clinical profession consist of duties to patients, duties to fellow professionals and duties to the general public. The fun-damental moral stricture from which ethical obligations arise is to place the needs of one's patients and fellow professionals before those of one-self.

All clinicians have, as a primary duty to their patients, to provide clinical services to the best of their abilities. In today's world, knowledge develops rapidly and the skills and understanding acquired as a student are quickly outdated. To fulfil their ethical obligations clinicians must constantly update their knowledge by continuing education and informed reading of the litera-ture. The possession of updated knowledge has the additional benefit that it increases confidence in one's ability, a confidence which transmits itself to the patient and inspires the trust which is the basis of a good professional relationship.

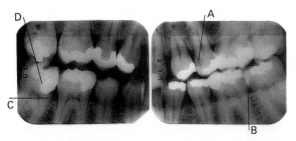

Figure 12.10   Bitewing radiographs showing approximal caries (A), approximal caries par-tially masked by overlapping contact area shadows (B), early bone loss due to periodontitis (C) and large restoration close to the pulp (D)

Apart from expecting a high standard of technical competence in the operator, patients expect to be treated safely. Instruments and equipment must be maintained so as to give their best performance, standards of cross-infection control must be rigorously applied, and the premises must conform to the appropriate health and safety regulations. In addition, clinicians must be careful about the way they dress. While it is unnecessary to adopt the manners and appearance of a bygone age, not all patients appreciate a flamboyant style. The elderly often associate such extremes of dress with antisocial behaviour and can take offence.

Patients also expect a degree of privacy during their treatment. This does not only mean that treatment should be performed out of sight and hearing of unwanted observers, but also that records which contain personal details must remain confidential. This applies to written and computer-based records. Both must be written up accurately and completely, and stored in a safe place protected from all except those with right of access.

Ethical obligations are not solely concerned with operator/patient relations. Clinicians also have obligations to their fellow professionals. The close personal relationship that clinicians establish with their patients is easily abused, the commonest way being by the criticism, actual or implied, of others. While we must always be truthful when dealing with patients, this can never be used as the opportunity to be judgemental.

Like dentists, dental hygienists are subject to regulations promulgated by the General Dental Council which govern the treatment they can provide. In due course it is likely that the duties of dental hygienists will evolve further. It is the ethical obligation of hygienists to conform to any regulations governing their registration, to know the limits to their duties, to be aware of any changes that might come about and to insist on the necessary level of support and supervision needed for them to carry out their duties adequately.

The final obligation is to the general public acting as tax payer. Dental treatment is expensive of time and materials. For those working in salaried posts it is especially difficult to be conscious of waste. Fine judgement is required if resources are not to be squandered on treatment of dental conditions with a poor prognosis, where treatment is provided more in hope than in the expectation of success.

Medical emergencies

The provision of treatment for dental patients involves working in the mouth, but it is most important that dental clinicians are aware of the fact that they are also responsible for the general well-being of the patient in the dental chair. Indeed, a responsibility exists until the patient has left the premises. An understanding of the medical emergencies that may occur together with their management is therefore important. A medical emergency may be of rapid onset, is quite often unexpected and requires immediate attention. The detection of a patient who may present with an acute medical problem begins as soon as the patient walks into the treatment room. Any new patient should be observed for signs of possible disease; these may include signs of pallor, which may indicate an underlying state of anaemia, or excessive stress or anxiety.

Breathlessness as a patient walks to the dental chair could indicate a cardiac or pulmonary condition. Careful checking of the medical history is important and it is recommended that all patients are questioned as to their current well-being by asking: 'Are you fit and healthy today?'. This may give a possible indication of whether an acute emergency could develop and allow adjustments of treatment to be made. These include having an oxygen supply near at hand, or only treating for a short time period. Pain control and/or sedation may be considered advisable when the level of anxiety is high. The commonest emergency which can occur in the dental chair is syncope (fainting) and the treatment of this will be covered first.

The first sign of a patient about to faint is pallor accompanied by a cold sweat and is often associated with a complaint of feeling dizzy, weak and nauseous. First aid should be given at once which includes laying the chair back so that the head is lower than the feet and loosening tight clothing. The radial pulse is weak and rapid. About 45 s later, as the blood flow to the brain begins to improve, the patient should start to feel better. Complete loss of consciousness can occur and any patient who has fainted should never be left unattended. This condition is not uncommon after giving a local anaesthetic, and for this reason the practice of returning the patient to the waiting room to allow the local anaesthetic to work is unsatisfactory.

Some patients respond poorly to the above treatment. A woman in the last 3 months of pregnancy should not be laid flat because the uterus will press on the inferior vena cava and reduce the venous return to the heart. Treatment is therefore given in the upright position and if she faints she should be placed on her side, care being taken to maintain the airway.

When consciousness returns, the patient may be given a glucose drink if they have missed a meal and, when they feel fit enough, treatment can continue. If signs of recovery are not evident after 45–60 s then the collapse may not be due to syncope. In this instance, the airway must be maintained, oxygen administered, and medical aid summoned.

Despite the most careful screening, a life-threatening emergency can still occur in patients undergoing dental treatment. Therefore all dental clinic personnel should be able to recognize the signs of a potential emergency and possess the skills to deal with it. The ability to carry out basic life support or cardiopulmonary resuscitation (CPR) is fundamental to this.

For dealing with emergencies that may occur in the dental surgery, the team approach is the most efficient. In a crisis, each member of the team assumes a specific duty. The team members should consider their educational background and skills and accept only the duties which they feel they can usefully perform. With the entire team trained in basic life support it should be possible to maintain a collapsed patient until medical help arrives. In most instances the dentist must accept a major role in the delivery of emergency care and responsibility for the administration of any drugs.

The emergency equipment available should include an oxygen supply and an emergency drug kit which may include the drugs listed in Table 12.1. The possible uses of oxygen in a medical emergency include the treatment of hypoxia and the establishment and maintenance of respiration. The

Table 12.1 The emergency drugs which should be available in an emergency kit

Drug	Indication	Dosage
Adrenaline (epinephrine)	Anaphylaxis	1 ml of 0.1% solution i.m. every 5 min
Hydrocortisone	Anaphylaxis or steroid crisis	Slow i.v. injection of 100 mg in 2 ml
Glyceryl trinitrate	Angina pectoris	0.4 mg tablet placed sublingually
Dextrose	Hypoglycaemia	50 mg dissolved in water
Atropine	Bradycardia	0.5 mg i.v.
Aminophylline	Asthma attack	0.5 gm i.v.
Diazepam	Status epilepticus	10 mg i.v.

A stethoscope and sphygmomanometer should be kept with the emergency drugs.

methods of oxygen delivery include exhaled air ventilation (as in CPR), atmospheric oxygen ventilation delivered by an Ambu bag and positive pressure oxygen ventilation from an oxygen cylinder. To ensure familiarity and confidence with emergency procedures the techniques should be regularly practised.

Signs of cardiorespiratory emergencies

Cardiac and respiratory arrest are two interrelated conditions. If either goes unrecognized or untreated it will rapidly progress to the other. The signs of cardiovascular failure may not be apparent until cardiac arrest or asystole occur. Pain may be felt in the chest which is commonly described as 'crushing' in nature. Patients showing these early signs must be allowed to adopt the position in which they feel most comfortable and initially treated as for fainting. If consciousness is lost they should be immediately laid flat and any tight clothing released, and the legs raised to improve venous blood return to the brain.

Should there be no improvement after 45 s then oxygen should be administered, and in the majority of cases recovery should occur. If the condition deteriorates further and there is loss of the carotid pulse and the patient becomes unrousable, CPR must be started. Respiratory arrest is usually preceded by depression of both rate and depth of respiration. Once this is recognized and providing breathing is still occurring, the administration of pure oxygen using a full face mask will usually effect recovery in 4–5 min. If breathing has stopped, then CPR is started.

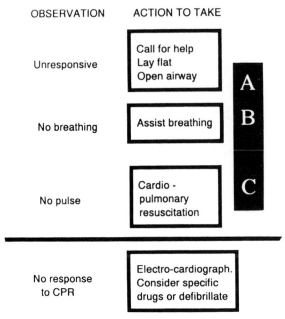

Figure 12.11   The ABC of cardiopulmonary resuscitation

Cardiopulmonary resuscitation (CPR)
The first step in CPR is to establish the state of consciousness of the patient. If there is no response to being spoken to or called, the patient is unconscious. Help should be sought and position the patient laid on a flat surface, preferably the floor. The ABC of CPR can then begin (Figure 12.11):

A for Airway. The airway should be opened using the head tilt-chin lift technique where the head is tilted back and the chin moves forward as in Figure 12.12. The mouth should be cleared of any foreign material or dentures, and a clear airway established.

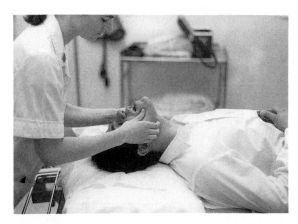

Figure 12.12   Establishing an adequate airway by pulling the mandible forward

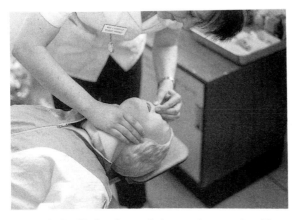

Figure 12.13 Closing the nasal airway prior to undertaking mouth-to-mouth resuscitation

B for Breathing. This is the restoration of lung inflation by artificial respiration (Figure 12.13).
C for Circulation. Establish if a carotid pulse is present (Figure 12.14). If a pulse is absent restore blood circulation by starting chest compressions.

The technique of CPR needs to be undertaken efficiently as time is of the essence. Permanent damage to the brain can occur if it is deprived of oxygen for longer than 3 min. Once the airway is clear and no breathing movements are seen, artificial respiration should begin. This is carried out by pinching the patient's nose, placing the operator's mouth over the patient's mouth and administering two slow but full breaths into the patient's lungs. If the idea of mouth-to-mouth contact is unpleasant, a lip seal can be maintained by placing two fingers across the lips. The patient's nose may then be used, and after placing the operator's mouth around it and achieving a lip seal, the

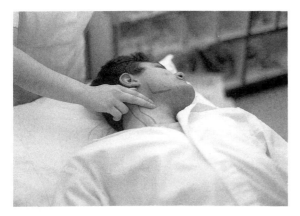

Figure 12.14 Check for the carotid pulse. This is felt beneath the angle of the mandible, in front of the sternomastoid muscle

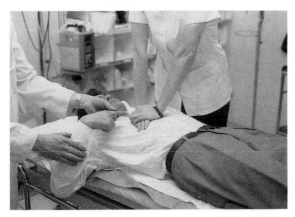

Figure 12.15   Undertake cardiac compression with the arms straight and the hands placed over the sternal notch

lungs can be inflated in a similar way. The movement of the chest is observed each time it is artificially inflated. After these initial two breaths, the carotid pulse should be checked. If a pulse is present in an adult, one new breath is given every 5 s amounting to 12/min. In a child one breath every 4 s or 15/min are required.

Should no pulse be detectable, external cardiac compression will be required. This involves correct positioning of the hands in the sternal notch which is located where the ribs meet the lower part of the sternum. The heel of the hand is placed into the area where compressions will begin and the other hand placed over it as in Figure 12.15. Compressions can begin with the intention of depressing the sternum between 1.5–2 inches in the adult, and 0.5–1 inches in a child aged 1–8 years (after this age adult compressions apply). If only one person is performing CPR, a ratio of 15 compressions to two breaths is administered and, to be effective, four cycles of 15:2 should be performed every minute.

When two people perform CPR one takes control of the chest compressions while the other establishes respiration. The technique is basically the same with two short breaths being administered initially to stimulate spontaneous breathing. The carotid pulse is then checked by the person giving 'mouth-to-mouth' and if this is absent the second person can begin chest compressions, five of which should be delivered before another breath is given by the first person. To establish a rhythm it is useful to count each chest compression aloud 'one, two, three, four, five and breathe'. The pulse should be checked every minute and the role of the two rescuers can be changed as tiredness sets in. CPR should be continued until expert medical help arrives (Figure 12.16).

Epilepsy

Fortunately most epileptics are well stabilized by regular drug therapy but occasionally, in a patient who is poorly stabilized, a grand mal seizure may occur. This can be frightening but there is usually an aura or premonition of

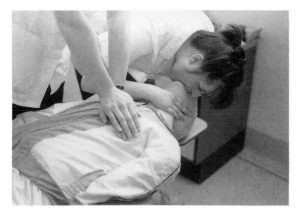

Figure 12.16   Cardiopulmonary resuscitation is possible in the dental chair

an impending attack, allowing dangerous objects to moved away. Good management involves preventing the patient injuring themselves during the attack and arranging for medical supervision and/or an escort home.

Allergic reactions

These may occur in response to local anaesthetics and can range from a skin rash to angio-oedema or circulatory collapse. Management is dependent on the severity of the symptoms.

Mild skin rashes which have developed over a day could be treated by an antihistamine such as terfenadine (Triludan), whereas a severe reaction involving the development of laryngeal oedema may require an intravenous injection of 100 mg hydrocortisone or an intramuscular administration of 0.5 ml of 0.1% adrenaline, prior to emergency hospital treatment.

Although an emergency arising in the dental surgery is a rare occurrence, it should be considered as a potential complication of treatment. Being able to recognize the patient who may present an emergency is important, but dealing with it effectively is critical.

Chapter 13

Complementary activities

Local analgesia

The effective control of pain for patients undergoing dental treatment is one of the major advances for the dental profession in the past 100 years. It is of vital importance that any clinician involved in the control of root surface deposits is very competent in its use.

The first record of a dental local analgesia being given in the UK was reported in the *Journal of the British Dental Association* in 1886 when William Hunt of Yeovil described the use of cocaine infiltrated into the tissues prior to dental treatment. Since then different local analgesia agents have been developed with lignocaine, which is the most widely used, being introduced into clinical practice in 1946. Subsequently two other drugs were developed, which are chemically related to lignocaine, namely mepivicaine (1956) and prilocaine (1959). Before considering the delivery and mode of action of these agents, it is worth revising the descriptive terminology which relates to pain, as well as how pain is produced.

Pain threshold

This refers to an individual's response to pain. One person may have a high pain threshold and therefore does not react to pain, whereas someone with a low threshold reacts violently to the mildest stimulus.

The pain threshold varies between individuals and can vary in the same person at different times.

Pain perception
This is the realization by the body that its tissues are at risk of damage.

Pain reaction
This is the interpretation of the pain stimulus which occurs in the cortex and posterior thalamus of the brain. A painful stimulus applied to different people will provide a range of responses. People who cry out when in pain are exhibiting the pain reaction.

Anatomical basis of dental pain

Stimuli which may produce an impulse in the nerve endings of the dental pulp or the supporting structures of the teeth are conveyed to the central nervous system by the second (maxillary) and the third (mandibular) divisions of the trigeminal nerve. From cell bodies in the Gasserian ganglion these neural pathways pass to the sensory nucleus of the trigeminal nerve which is situated in the medulla oblongata. They then pass into the thalamus where they are relayed via connecting neurones to the cortex of the brain on the opposite side of the body from where the original stimulus arose.

Local analgesia: general considerations

The use of local analgesia has made the delivery of dental treatment much easier for both clinician and patient. There are comparatively few contraindications to the use of local analgesic agents and in the case of infiltration local analgesia the working time in most patients should be up to three-quarters of an hour. Those circumstances when the use of local analgesia must be carefully considered are as follows:

1. The presence of acute infection at the operative site which may be exacerbated by injecting into the area.
2. In patients who possess a bleeding diathesis such as haemophilia or von Willebrand's disease. In these patients excess bleeding from the injection site can occur unless they have been specifically covered for dental treatment by a haematologist before any care is delivered.
3. Some authorities advise caution when using a local anaesthetic in patients who suffer from cardiovascular disease. This relates to the presence of adrenaline in the anaesthetic solution which can be injected intravascularly – an event which tends to occur more frequently when giving mandibular block injections and can be avoided by using an aspirating syringe. Alternatively a local analgesic can be used which contains no vasoconstrictor.
4. Some patients report hypersensitivity to the commonly used agents but this is rare and other alternatives are available.
5. The use of a local analgesic containing a vasoconstrictor in patients who have had radiotherapy to the area around the mouth is to be discouraged due to the possibility of introducing infection into an area which already has decreased vascularity. A local analgesic without vasoconstrictor may be suitable if the patient's consultant radiotherapist approves the use of local analgesia.

Types of local analgesia

The types of local analgesia which can be used may be categorized according to the point at which the agent acts. Surface or topical analgesia is when the anaesthetic is applied to the surface mucosa for blocking superficial nerve endings in the mucous membrane. Infiltration analgesia is when the anaesthetic is placed into the connective tissue where it can infiltrate through the tissues to block nerve impulses locally. Regional analgesia is when a nerve trunk is blocked so that an area of the body is rendered numb.

Mode of action

All local analgesic agents are formed from a weak base and a strong acid. They are readily broken down in human tissues to liberate an alkaloid compound which is then free to be taken up by the lipids in the axon. As the hydrochloride salt is the most common form in which the agent is used, the process may be represented by the following equation:

$$B\ HCl + NaHCO_3 \rightarrow B + NaCl + H_2CO_3$$
$$\text{(free base)}$$

The precise mode of action of the free base (B) is not known but it would appear to prevent the increase in sodium permeability of the nerve membrane and hence block the transmission of an impulse along the axon. The propagation of a nerve impulse under normal conditions is shown in Figure 13.1.

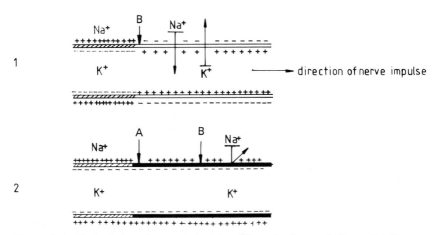

Figure 13.1 Transmission of a nerve impulse: (1) a stimulus applied at point B causes depolarization of the axon allowing sodium and potassium ions to move in the direction shown; (2) when a local anaesthetic drug is present at point A the movement of sodium and potassium ions is prevented so that no nerve impulse is generated

Contents of a local analgesic cartridge

The local analgesic cartridge as used in dentistry has six constituents:

1. Local analgesic solution, most commonly 2% lignocaine hydrochloride.

2. Vasoconstrictor, 1:80 000 adrenaline.
3. Reducing agent (sodium metabisulphite) to prevent the oxidation of the vasoconstrictor.
4. Preservative (caprylhydrocuprienotoxin) to maintain shelf life for up to 2 years.
5. Fungicide (thymol) to stop the solution becoming cloudy.
6. The vehicle (modified Ringer's solution) in which the above compounds are dissolved.

Infiltration local analgesia

For the purposes of scaling sensitive teeth and root planing, infiltration analgesia is normally all that is required, but on occasions mandibular teeth will still be sensitive and so a mandibular block injection will be required. Prior to the injection of the local analgesic agent a topical analgesic may be used to anaesthetize superficial nerve endings in the mucous membrane. This may be particularly indicated in the maxillary anterior region where the administration of an injection into the vestibule can be quite uncomfortable for the patient. This surface preparation is also advisable when the palatal tissues are to be anaesthetized. Topically applied agents can be obtained in the form of a spray which contains 10% lignocaine hydrochloride in a water miscible base, or in the form of an ointment which contains 5% lignocaine hydrochloride which is applied on a cotton wool roll 3–4 min before giving the injection. Topical analgesia is not always required, but in some patients it can be helpful, particularly if they are anxious.

When a local analgesic infiltration is given the solution is placed into the tissues above the periosteum. A painless, efficient technique should be used and every precaution taken to avoid complications. The commonest complication of administering a local analgesic is that of the patient fainting. It is almost impossible for the patient to faint if they are in the supine position in the dental chair and so it is recommended, where possible, to put the chair back into this position. The loading of the syringe is accomplished in the normal way, but it is worthwhile to restate that a new needle should be used each time and a cartridge that has already been used but still contains some solution must never be reused.

Technique of injection
Before proceeding with the injection it is worthwhile to have a pair of artery forceps to hand in case the needle breaks in the tissues. This is an extremely rare occurrence nowadays, but if it did happen the needle could be removed from the tissues while still visible. If a broken needle is not removed immediately, it will rapidly submerge and as a result have to be removed surgically.

The stages of injection are as follows:

1. Examine the proposed injection site and make sure there are no signs of infection or ulceration. Dry the surface mucosa with a cotton wool roll. Some authorities recommend the application of an antiseptic solution

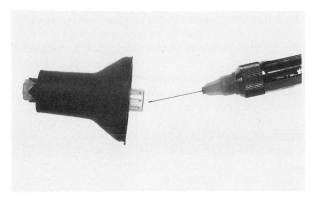

Figure 13.2   The needle is inspected prior to use

such as cetrimide, on a cotton wool roll, to clean the mucosa before it is punctured by the needle.
2. Remove the needle guard and eject a small amount of solution to check that the needle is not blocked and at the same time check the needle point to make sure it is sharp (Figure 13.2).
3. Pull the surface mucosa taut so that the tissues will be easily penetrated by the needle and as soon as the needle has penetrated the tissue inject a little solution so that a small blister is raised just under the surface (Figure 13.3). Wait a few seconds before advancing a few millimetres further into the tissue. Inject the main bulk of solution after the tension in the tissues has been relaxed. Inject about 0.5 ml of solution for each tooth to be anaesthetized. This technique can be used for all injections into the maxillary or mandibular vestibule.

Anaesthesia of palatal tissues
An injection into the palatal tissues is more difficult because the mucoperiosteum is of firm consistency and tightly bound down to bone except at the

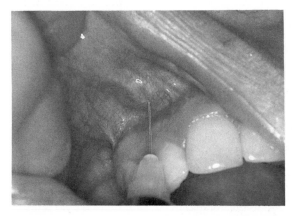

Figure 13.3   A small 'bleb' is raised under the mucosa when giving a buccal local anaesthetic infiltration

angle between the horizontal aspect of the palate and the alveolus. Even there the small amount of distensible tissue means that a greater pressure is required when injecting the solution than is necessary in other areas. As a palatal infiltration can be uncomfortable for the patient, the initial application of topical analgesic is recommended. The site of the injection should be about 1 cm away from the free gingival margin where the tissue will be a little thicker and, as a result, can more easily accommodate the small amount of anaesthetic solution needed. Care should be taken not to inject too close to the palatine foramen as this will result in the lesser palatine nerve being affected. Anaesthesia of the soft palate can develop and cause distress to the patient by causing difficulty in swallowing. For this reason it is recommended that palatal injections are never given posterior to the second molar tooth. The amount of solution to inject for a single palatal injection should be just enough to induce localized raising of the tissue; the volume of solution needed to produce this is about 0.5 ml.

Anaesthesia in the mandible
Buccal infiltration analgesia in the mandible is essentially the same as that for the maxillary buccal injection. If a lingual infiltration is necessary, then the injection is made into the mucosa as it reflects from the floor of mouth mucosa to alveolar mucosa as in Figure 13.4. Careful tongue retraction using a dental mirror aids positioning of the needle which on puncturing the mucous membrane only needs to pass about 3–4 mm into the tissues before the solution is injected. The volume of solution required to produce anaesthesia of the lingual gingival tissues is again no more than 0.5 ml.

The inferior alveolar block
By blocking the inferior alveolar and lingual nerves on one side together with the long buccal nerve where necessary, a more prolonged and effective level of local analgesia may be obtained. A 27 gauge needle is used which is 3.5 cm long, the depth of penetration into the tissues being about 2.5 cm. Prior to inserting the needle the anatomical landmarks must be identified. This begins by placing the thumb of the hand which is not holding the syringe on the external oblique ridge of the mandible. The deepest concavity of the

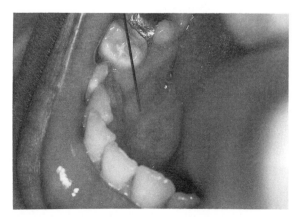

Figure 13.4   The position for a mandibular lingual infiltration in the premolar region

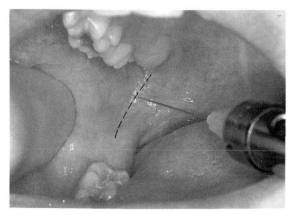

Figure 13.5 The line traces the path of the pterygomandibular raphe. The needle passes buccally to this

ridge is palpated. The next structure to identify is the pterygomandibular raphe, the approximate position of which is illustrated in Figure 13.5. The needle is inserted just beneath the mucosa at a point which bisects the thumb nail and lies just to the outer or lateral aspect of the pterygomandibular raphe. A small amount of local analgesic is injected. With the barrel of the syringe held parallel to the mandibular occlusal plane and lying over the second premolar of the opposite side of the mouth, the needle is advanced further for about 0.5 cm and about a fifth of the cartridge contents is injected to anaesthetize the lingual nerve. The needle can then be advanced a further 1.5–2.0 cm until it lightly contacts the bone of the inner aspect of the mandible (Figure 13.6). It is then withdrawn slightly and three-fifths of the cartridge contents are injected, leaving a small amount of anaesthetic solution in the syringe which can then be withdrawn completely. The remaining solution can be used to anaesthetize the long buccal nerve which curves around the distal aspect of the last molar tooth. The needle is inserted just under the mucosa where it will hit bone at once. It is withdrawn very slightly

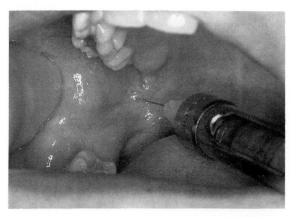

Figure 13.6 The needle position when giving an inferior alveolar block local anaesthetic injection

and the remaining solution injected. A satisfactory level of mandibular anaesthesia should be obtained within 3–4 min.

Difficulties and complications of local analgesia

The widespread use of local analgesia in both medical and dental practice is an indication of its value and safety, but there are various difficulties and complications that can be experienced when it is used. Those of particular importance may be listed as follows:

Local
1. Pain on injection.
2. Haematoma formation.
3. Intravascular injection.
4. Blanching of tissue.
5. Lip trauma.
6. Needle track infection.
7. Visual disturbance.
8. Broken needle.

General
1. Anxiety.
2. Fainting (syncope).
3. Adverse drug reaction.
4. Cardiorespiratory effects.

Pain during or after injection
A considerable number of patients are anxious about all forms of dental treatment, with the dental local anaesthetic injection producing most anxiety. To reduce anxiety when giving dental injections, a sympathetic attitude is as important as gentle technique. Most infiltrations given buccally are virtually painless if the tissues are stretched prior to inserting the needle and the solution injected slowly with minimal force. Pain several hours later after the anaesthetic effect has dissipated could be due to infection or haematoma formation.

Haematoma formation
This occasionally develops after an infiltration if the needle has passed through a superficial blood vessel, so allowing excess bleeding to occur into the tissues. It should not be a problem with buccally placed infiltrations, but if a palatal injection traumatizes the greater palatine vessels as a result of the needle being inserted too high in the palatal vault, postoperative swelling and pain may result.

Intravascular injection
To avoid the complication of an intravascular injection an aspirating syringe should be used. The signs of an intravascular injection are similar to those of

a faint which are described in Chapter 12. When this happens the procedure should be abandoned and the patient placed in the supine position and carefully supervised until full recovery.

Blanching
Blanching at the site of the injection is not unusual and is produced by the vasoconstrictor in the solution. When blanching occurs at a site more distant it may be due to an intravascular injection or interference with the autonomic nerve supply to local blood vessels. Providing the infiltration is not given too deeply, blanching of distant tissues such as the cheeks should not occur.

Lip trauma
This can be caused by the operator, accidentally by the patient, or deliberately as a result of the patient testing a still numb lip to see if the sensation is returning (usually by biting it).

Needle track infection
This is a rare complication now that pre-sterilized disposable equipment is used.

Visual disturbance
This is fortunately a rare complication and is due to intra-arterial injection producing ocular vascular spasm. Normal vision should be restored within 30 min but it is worthwhile in these days of increasing litigation to seek an opinion from an ophthalmic surgeon if there is any doubt about recovery.

Broken needle
This is also rare as needles are only used once. However, it is recommended to have a pair of artery forceps in a nearby drawer just in case the impossible happens. The end remaining outside the tissues can be readily seized.

The general complications which may be seen as a result of receiving a local anaesthetic are covered in the section on Medical Emergencies.

Rubber dam application

All too often dental procedures are carried out on teeth contaminated by saliva and plaque, and soon after the start of operative procedures there is additional contamination by blood and crevicular fluid. Ideally all procedures should be carried out on clean dry teeth. Such conditions are especially difficult for the periodontist or hygienist to achieve, who when carrying out procedures such as root planing finds it impossible to avoid damage to the gingivae at all times. Nevertheless, while conventional moisture control procedures can be very effective for procedures such as prophylaxis, scaling and root planing, for other procedures higher standards are needed.

The ideal method of moisture control is application of rubber dam, a method obligatory in endodontics where it gives the additional advantages of preventing cross-infection and protecting the patient's airway. Rubber dam is useful at many other times, however, because all dental materials give optimal results when used under the kind of conditions which resemble the laboratories in which they were developed. When amalgam is contaminated by moisture during use it becomes liable to corrosion and excessive expansion. Contaminated composite resins show diminished adhesion, microleakage and discolouration. The surface integrity of glass ionomer cements is affected by moisture changes in their environment and their adhesion to teeth is reduced by saliva contamination at insertion. Finally, application of desensitizing agents, dentine bonding agents and topical fluorides is more effective (and safer) in the absence of saliva contamination, and set restorations can be polished to a higher standard.

Rubber dam is helpful in other ways apart from preventing moisture contamination. It protects the working field, the operator and the operator's instruments from contamination by the patient's oral flora and is especially indicated for patients with diseases such as hepatitis B where cross-infection is a great danger. Rubber dam also acts as a physical barrier, protecting the patient's tongue and cheeks from damage by rotating or sharp instruments, and when working with small instruments rubber dam effectively guards the airway and digestive tract against their inhalation or ingestion. These advantages far outweigh any possible disadvantages which may include a reduction in the amount of communication possible and an occasional complaint of claustrophobia. Residues of the chemicals used in the processing of latex may also produce an allergic response in a very small number of patients.

Equipment

The rubber dam itself is a thin sheet of latex which forms a watertight junction around the cervical margin of the tooth so excluding moisture from the operative field. The necessary equipment for its application includes a rubber dam punch and frame, rubber dam forceps, an assortment of clamps and a supply of waxed floss silk (Figure 13.7). A lubricant, most conveniently topical anaesthetic gel, is useful for helping the rubber dam pass through tight interdental contacts.

Rubber dam is generally supplied in 6-inch black or green squares of which medium thickness is the most popular. More recently it has become available in a range of pastel shades and pleasant tastes. At an appropriate place a hole is punched in the dam through which the selected tooth crown passes, so isolating the tooth from the rest of the mouth. Until experience is acquired a rubber dam stamp is useful and serves to premark the dam with the sites of teeth in their arches. Once applied, then provided that the punched hole is narrower in diameter than the cervical margin of the tooth, the dam will be retained mechanically. For most procedures the dam at the cervical margin of the tooth is encouraged to enter the gingival crevice, so exposing the maximum clinical crown. If desired the edge of the dam can be inverted into place with a small flat plastic instrument.

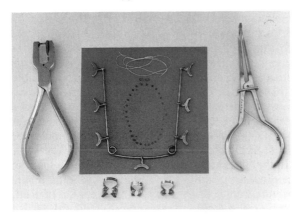

Figure 13.7   Rubber dam equipment including punch, forceps, sheet of rubber dam, floss silk, Fernauld frame and selection of clamps

While rubber dam punches and forceps are of standard form, rubber dam frames are of two types. The original metal Fernauld frame is a U-shaped piece of thick wire to which the dam was attached by being stretched over short T-bars extending outwards. More modern forms are made of plastic and the dam is attached by stretching it over short 'spikes' protruding from the periphery.

Rubber dam clamps consist of two blades engaging the cervical margin of the tooth and joined by a connector of springy steel. They are of various sizes depending on the tooth they are to be attached to (Figure 13.8). Rubber dam clamps do not always fit precisely and in general we have to be satisfied with two-point contact between the blade and the tooth. Where only one-point contact exists the blade can be narrowed and adjusted with a mounted carborundum disc. When repeatedly trying in clamps to check their fit, secure them with a piece of floss silk – clamps have been known to fracture in use. Depending on whether the edge of the blade is straight or curved

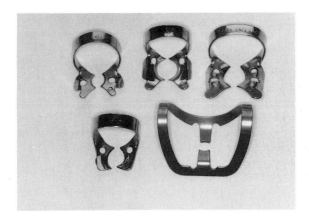

Figure 13.8   Selection of rubber dam clamps, including: (a) winged premolar clamp; (b) and (c) two sizes of winged molar clamps with blades curved to enter gingival crevice; (d) small wingless clamp for molar or premolar; (e) Ferrier clamp for anterior teeth

downwards to enter the gingival crevice, the clamp will be suitable for fully erupted or partly erupted teeth.

On the clamp, next to the blades, are found points of attachment – either holes or notches – for the rubber dam forceps, and using these the clamp is applied to the tooth and removed afterwards. Most clamps also possess small projections or wings which serve for temporary attachment of the dam to the clamp during its manipulation outside the mouth. They are found adjacent to the site of application of the forceps. As mentioned above, rubber dam clamps have been known to fracture and hence should not be placed in the mouth unless secured with floss silk or first attached by their wings to the rubber dam. In the latter case, if the clamp then fractures while being placed, the broken pieces will remain external to the mouth and cannot be ingested or inhaled. Wingless clamps are available and are used, after initial application of the dam, to improve access by securing the dam to more distal teeth. Extra holes are then unnecessary.

Application

The method of application of rubber dam varies slightly according to the number and type of teeth to be isolated and methods appropriate to each will be described. Prior to any attempt to apply rubber dam, however, any interproximal contacts through which the dam must pass are tested for patency with waxed floss silk.

Application to a single molar or premolar tooth
A sheet of rubber dam is selected and a hole punched in the appropriate place using one of the larger guides on the punch. Sometimes, for large molars, two interconnected holes are needed. A suitably sized, winged clamp is chosen and placed in the punched hole retaining the dam on the clamp wings, with the connector posteriorly. After the frame has in turn been attached to the dam, the clamp is engaged by the forceps (Figure 13.9) and the entire assembly picked up and placed on the tooth (Figure 13.10).

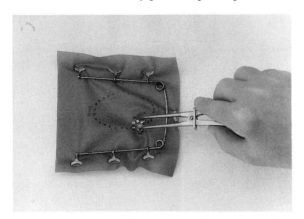

Figure 13.9   Dam in place on frame, clamp connected to dam by wings, and forceps engaged in clamp prior to placing assembly in mouth

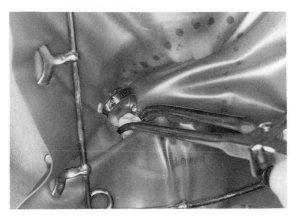

Figure 13.10   United dam, frame and clamp placed on tooth

When the clamp is secure the dam is slipped from the wings to seal the cervical margin (Figure 13.11). After completing the dental procedure the rubber dam is removed after first removing the clamp.

Application to a single anterior tooth
A hole is again punched at the appropriate place in the rubber dam and the sheet of dam attached to the frame. The tissue side of the hole in the dam is lubricated with a small amount of topical anaesthetic gel and the dam placed in position over the tooth, passing the edge of the dam through the interdental contacts. To ensure that the sheet of rubber dam is retained on the tooth and that the edge of the dam enters, and is retained in the gingival crevice, a floss silk ligature is applied. A piece of waxed silk approximately 25 cm long is passed twice round the tooth. Holding the free ends firmly in one hand and using a small flat plastic instrument, the ligature is pushed down to the cervical margin of the tooth, carrying the dam with it. Once the ligature is sufficiently far cervically it will be retained at the narrowest point of the tooth and is secured by a double hitch.

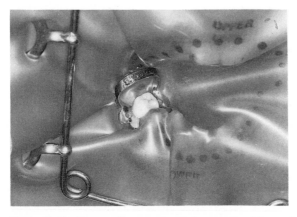

Figure 13.11   Forceps disengaged and dam removed from wings in order to secure seal at cervical margin of tooth

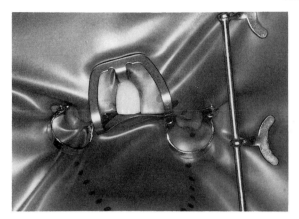

Figure 13.12   Dam secured on maxillary central incisor by means of a Ferrier clamp and access enhanced by further clamps on the premolars

Alternatively a clamp can be used. After placing the dam on the tooth by hand it is drawn up with the fingers to expose the cervical margin, at which point a clamp is applied. A Ferrier type clamp is the most useful.

Whichever method is used, for further security and improved access the dam can be held down by clamps in the premolar region. Small, winged or wingless clamps are applied to a premolar tooth, on each side, over the dam. It is unnecessary to punch a hole beforehand (Figure 13.12).

Application to several posterior teeth
A number of holes are punched in the dam according to the site and number of the teeth to be isolated. For best access include, if possible, the tooth distal to the operative site. As before, a clamp is engaged into the most distal hole, by its wings, and the frame attached to the dam periphery. After lubricating the internal surface of the punched holes, the clamp, frame and related dam are applied to the tooth, the dam freed from the clamp wings and pushed down over the crowns of the teeth to be isolated, each in its appropriate hole. Floss silk is used to pass the lubricated dam through the contacts. If, after application, the dam does not pass immediately into the gingival crevice it can be inverted into place with a flat plastic instrument.

To improve access a clamp can be applied over a tooth on the contralateral side (Figure 13.13). Where lip activity is marked and it is feared that it might displace the dam, a further clamp can be applied over the dam, on the same side, but anterior to the site of operation.

Application to several anterior teeth
The ligature method is used as for application to a single anterior tooth. The correct number of holes are punched and after the teeth have been pushed through the dam, small wingless clamps are applied over the premolar teeth in order to secure the dam firmly before ligatures are applied. When the dam is fully in place, ligatures are applied to all isolated teeth (Figures 13.14 and

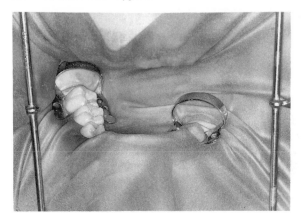

Figure 13.13 Access to isolated mandibular teeth improved by placing a clamp over a contralateral premolar

13.15). By inserting wedges interdentally, additional security is given for ensuring that the dam remains in the gingival crevice.

Removal of rubber dam

To remove the dam all retaining clamps, ligatures and wedges are removed. If a single tooth has been isolated the dam can then be drawn away from the crown. When several teeth have been isolated the dam may still resist removal. The dam is then pulled buccally or labially away from the cervical margins of the teeth and the connections between the punched holes cut with scissors, taking care to avoid damage to the lips or cheeks.

Special situations

When uncontaminated access to the cervical margin of a tooth is essential

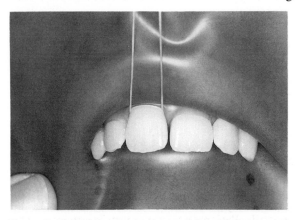

Figure 13.14 Rubber dam in place and floss silk ligature being applied to maxillary central incisor

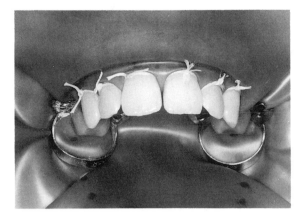

Figure 13.15 Floss silk ligatures applied to all maxillary anterior teeth and dam secured by premolar clamps

some degree of gingival retraction may be needed, typically where a caries or abrasion lesion extends to the gingival margin and a restoration or desensitizing material is to be applied. A cervical clamp is then useful. The most popular is the Ferrier clamp. This is characterized by two narrow connectors, one on either side of the blades, each of which is notched for attachment of the forceps (Figures 13.8). The shape of the connectors is such as to make access to the tooth easier from the buccal side (Figure 13.12). The blades are narrow and sharp and the labial is bent to enter the gingival crevice and contact the tooth 1 mm or so apical to the lingual contact. The sharp blades ensure firm attachment to the tooth but attempts to place the labial blade further apically than the lingual blade by more than 1 mm or so will lead only to instability of the clamp or damage to the lingual gingival margin.

If ever a bridge has to be involved in the rubber dam, application is more difficult. Holes are punched as normal but those holes related to the bridge abutments are joined by a scissors cut. The rubber dam will now fit over the bridge and protect the airway but unfortunately some moisture contamination can occur from the gingival crevice. Because the attachment is relatively less secure, application of clamps on either side of the bridge is advisable.

Final points

Although the application of rubber dam is a painless procedure in the hands of a skilled operator, some discomfort can arise if it is to be in place for longer than a few minutes. To prevent maceration of the skin after the dam has been applied, a conventional saliva ejector should be inserted and dental napkins placed between the patient's lips and the edges of the dam.

Some interference with breathing can occur and it is best to cut away the dam around the patient's nostrils. Patients who are mouth breathers may be inconvenienced if there is a good seal between the lips and the dam. To aid breathing in such cases, accessory holes can be cut in the upper part of the dam, but ensure that none is as large as the smallest instrument to be used.

Impressions and study models

Well made study models are useful to the dental health worker. They provide a teaching aid to which a patient can relate personally and are an accurate measure of the progress of tooth surface loss (Figure 13.16).

Materials

Impressions for study models are taken in stock trays (Figure 13.17) using an alginate impression material. Although plastic disposable trays are available, the best stock trays are of metal. They are produced in a range of sizes and are nickel plated to reduce corrosion. The correct size is chosen after first measuring with dividers the width of the dental arch in the canine and molar region and comparing this with the selected tray. To ensure that the set impression material is securely attached to the tray, a perforated tray is preferred. In the absence of perforations the tray is given a thin coating of tray adhesive.

Alginate is a hydrocolloid extracted from seaweed. It is supplied as a fine powder comprising a soluble alginate salt (either sodium or potassium) and filler (diatomaceous earth). When mixed with water it forms a smooth paste which sets after a few minutes to form a tough elastic gel. The setting reaction is of interest and provides an excellent example of how the applied scientist can modify chemical reactions so that material properties conform to clinical requirements. To ensure that the mixed paste sets, the powder formulation includes a calculated amount of calcium carbonate and, as it

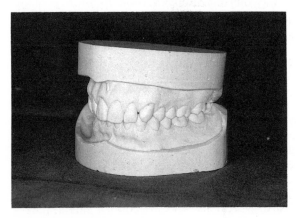

Figure 13.16   Plaster models

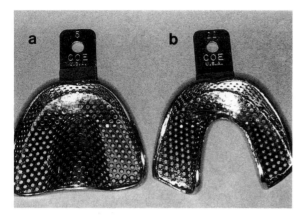

Figure 13.17   Perforated, metal stock trays: (a) upper; (b) lower

slowly dissolves in the mixing water, calcium ions are released which sub-stitute for the sodium or potassium ions of the alginate salt. Calcium being divalent, the reaction cross-links the polymer chains to form a three-dimensional network. To prevent the reaction occurring too quickly and to allow adequate time for thorough mixing, a further small calculated amount of sodium phosphate is also included. The calcium ions which are first released then react preferentially with the sodium phosphate to form very insoluble calcium phosphate. This gives a minute or so of delay while the sodium phosphate is used up, so that thorough mixing can take place before setting begins.

Technique

Before mixing alginate the container in which it is supplied is inverted once or twice to mix the powder and prevent settling. If left unused for a while, water vapour from the atmosphere reacts with surface powder and if the surface is not disturbed regularly the setting reaction will be inconsistent. For the same reason a small residue in a large tin of alginate should be discarded.

Alginate powder should be dispensed exactly according to the manufac-turer's instructions, taking care not to pack down the powder into its measure otherwise extra alginate will be included and the mixture will be too stiff to use. After mixing, the alginate is loaded into the tray and the surface smoothed with a wet finger. Maxillary impressions are taken with the operator standing or sitting behind the patient (Figure 13.18) and the patient's head at chest level. Using the fingers of the spare hand to retract the lips the tray is introduced into the mouth and seated first over the anterior teeth. When the tray is accurately sited it is rotated up at the back to seat over the posterior teeth. In this way defects in the centre of the palate will be avoided. Mandibular impressions are taken with the operator in front of the patient (Figure 13.19). The entire arch will be visible and the tray can be

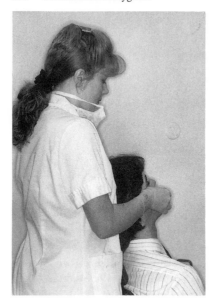

Figure 13.18   Correct operator position for maxillary impression

accurately and evenly sited before being depressed into position. As the tray is seated the patient is asked to protrude the tongue. This ensures that the impression material enters the lingual sulcus and prevents the lateral margins of the tongue being trapped.

The mouth is a complex structure and there are normally undercuts to be recorded, both of soft tissue and hard tissue. Hence to remove the set material it has to be distorted to some extent. All set elastomeric impression materials are visco-elastic and, when distorted by removal from an under-cut, require time to resume their original shape. For optimum accuracy the period of distortion should be as short as possible, and the period of recovery prolonged. Impressions are, therefore, removed from the mouth with a jerk, warning the patient beforehand. Before being cast they are checked to ensure that all the teeth and the related sulci are recorded (Figure 13.20), then left for a period of about 15 min for elastic recovery to take place.

Disinfection

Before casting, impressions are held under running water to remove traces of mucus and blood before being placed in a 1% solution of hypochlorite for 5 min. Some makes of alginate do not withstand this regime well and suffer surface deterioration. A preliminary check should be made that the alginate used is suitable for this method of disinfection. As an alternative, after washing as before, the impression and tray can be sprayed with a hard-surface antiseptic.

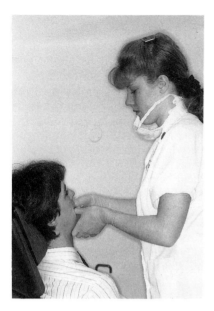

Figure 13.19   Correct operator position for mandibular impression

Following the recommended period of immersion the impression is again rinsed in water to remove excess hypochlorite. It is important that the period of immersion is not too prolonged. Being a hydrocolloid, alginate will gain or lose water from the environment and change shape accordingly. Long periods of immersion in water cause the material to expand, and if left in dry air it will shrink.

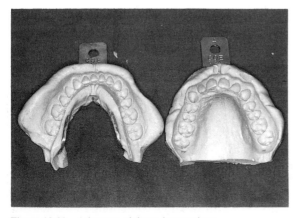

Figure 13.20   Adequate alginate impressions

Casting

Alginate impressions must be cast soon after being taken. If they are to be transported or kept for casting at a later time they must be placed in a sealable polythene bag and protected against contact with hard surfaces.

Impressions are cast in plaster of Paris, dental stone or a mixture of the two. In the manufacture of plaster of Paris, calcium sulphate dihydrate is converted into its hemihydrate by heat. Simple heating in air produces a white powder (plaster of Paris) with large amorphous crystals. Heating with superheated steam produces a yellowish powder consisting of small crystals (dental stone). Adding water rehydrates the powder and converts it back into the hemihydrate, a small amount of heat being liberated. Both plaster and stone are used for the casting of impressions but the small crystals of dental stone can be mixed to a workable consistency with a smaller amount of water. Consequently, when mixed to similar consistencies and allowed to set, a model cast from plaster of Paris contains more water and is much weaker than one cast from a dental stone. For most purposes a compromise may be made and the impression cast using a 50:50 (w/w) mixture of plaster and stone.

To the appropriate amount of water in a bowl, plaster is added gradually, taking care not to incorporate air, until with minimum stirring a workable consistency is produced. A little is then poured into the impression and vibrated so that it runs into the impressions of the teeth without including air bubbles. When the impression has been filled by successive additions it is inverted onto a mound of plaster and allowed to set. When the plaster has fully set (detectable by the exothermic heat of setting) the tray can be carefully removed and the base and sides of the model trimmed to the conventional shape. Finally, small pimples of excess plaster are removed from the tissue surface of the model with a sharp knife.

If a model is to be kept for some considerable time it is advantageous to harden the surface to resist abrasion and a coating of surface-hardening resin is recommended. The appearance of such models is also better if, instead of the base being formed freehand, the impressions are inverted into base pre-forms of plastic.

Pack and suture removal

Although during the past 10 years there has been a rapid decline in the amount of periodontal surgery performed there are still circumstances where the use of a pack may be necessary, for example after a gingivectomy. In this circumstance a periodontal dressing is placed at the time of completion of surgery and it is left in place for a period of 1 week. The types of periodontal dressing available can be divided into those that contain Eugenol and those that do not. The most commonly used are the non-Eugenol dressings and examples of these include Coe-pak (Coe Laboratories, Chicago, Illinois) and Peri-pac (de Trey Freres S.A., Zurich, Switzerland). The constituents of these dressings vary with Coe-pak containing zinc oxide, an oil for plasticity, a gum for cohesiveness and lorothidol (a fungicide). Peri-pac contains fatty acids derived from coconut oil in liquid form, which are thickened with colophony resin and includes chlorothymol (a bacteriostatic agent).

When the patient returns for a review appointment the dressing will require removal and this is easily accomplished by placing a flat plastic instrument under one area of the dressing and gently easing it away from the teeth. This should enable the dressing to be removed in one piece. The gingival tissues underneath will be covered with a white slough which is made up of desquamated epithelial cells, micro-organisms and elements of dental plaque.

It is advisable to remove this slough gently using a cotton wool pledget soaked in chlorhexidine. Depending on the progress of healing a new dressing may be required for a further week or the area left uncovered, in which case modified plaque removal instructions are given, to include the use of a soft brush, together with regular chlorhexidine rinsing.

If flap surgery has been performed and sutures have been placed to secure wound closure, these are usually left in place for 7 days. Suture materials can be absorbable or non-absorbable. Examples of absorbable sutures include plain gut which is prepared from the submucosa of sheep intestine, and synthetic chromic gut. Non-absorbable sutures include silk, cotton and synthetic sutures and these will definitely require removal. Absorbable sutures can take in excess of 10 days to be absorbed and so, if they are found to still be in place after 7 days, are removed at the review appointment for the patient's comfort.

Removing sutures is very easy and the following approach is recommended. Prior to removal the sutures should be swabbed with chlorhexidine to reduce the bacterial contamination. The patient's record should be consulted to see how many sutures were placed at the end of the operation and a check made to see how many are still present in the mouth, as some may have been lost during the healing period. The suture knot is then grasped with College forceps and the suture lifted just sufficiently to allow the open points of small suture scissors to be inserted around the suture before it enters the gingival tissue. The suture is cut cleanly, then gently removed and placed on a tissue. All remaining sutures are removed in a similar fashion so that a final count can be made on completion.

If a continuous suture has been placed it must not be removed by drawing it through the tissue. In this case all the vertical loops are cut as they enter the tissue and these are individually removed in a similar way to that of the single sutures. After suture removal, advice on plaque control procedures in the surgical area should be given to the patient. This should involve gentle flossing and brushing combined with chlorhexidine rinsing for a further 2 weeks. A review appointment is arranged for a few weeks' time when healing should be complete. Pocket depths may be checked by probing with a periodontal probe 6 weeks after surgery.

Appendix: Disease assessment

Periodontal assessment forms

There are two main methods of periodontal charting forms in use: pictorial and numerical. The pictorial forms have diagrams of the teeth on which the relevant details can be superimposed. A typical form is reproduced in Figure A.1. The numerical chart relies on a straightforward listing of the details.

PERIODONTAL EXAMINATION CHART

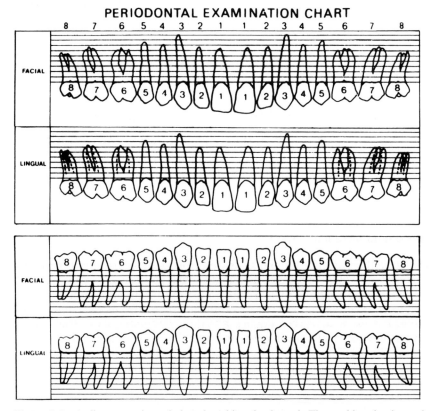

Figure A.1 A diagrammatic periodontal probing depth card. The probing depth can be reproduced on the millimetre markings overlying the stylised teeth diagrams

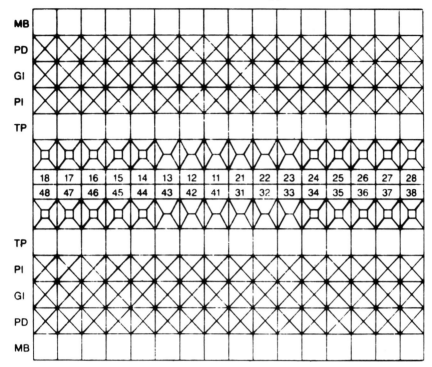

Figure A.2   A numerical periodontal chart. This particular variation allows four or six point charting

Although the former diagrammatic type would seem to give useful information, because periodontal monitoring relies upon the gathering of information over a long period of time, the authors would recommend the numerical type shown in Figure A.2. However, both are reproduced here so readers can make up their own minds on the most useful method.

Periodontal screening system

The Basic Periodontal Examination described here is based on the Community Periodontal Index of Treatment Needs, as amended by the working party of the British Society of Periodontology (BSP) and first produced in their policy statement – *Periodontology in General Dental Practice in the United Kingdom*, and is reproduced with their kind permission. The authors have made some minor changes from the BSP document and these are indicated by italics.

For the periodontal examination the dentition is divided into six sextants, as shown in Figure A.3.

The use of a periodontal probe is mandatory. The recommended probe is the *World Health Organization probe which has a ball end 0.5 mm diameter. A colour coded area extends from 3.5 mm to 5.5 mm. A newer version of the*

WHO probe has a second dark band running from 8.5 to 11.5 mm, as shown in Figure 12.1, to assist in estimating the depth of very deep pockets. Probing force should not exceed 20–25 g.

The probe tip is gently inserted into the gingival pocket and the depth of insertion read against the colour coding. The total extent of the pocket should be explored, conveniently by 'walking' the probe around the pocket. At least six points on each tooth should be examined: mesiobuccal, mid-buccal, distobuccal and the corresponding lingual sites.

For each sextant the highest score *together with an * if appropriate* is recorded. A sextant with only one tooth is recorded as missing and the score is included in the adjacent sextant. A simple box is used to record the scores for each sextant as shown in Figure A.3. *The following codings are used:*

Code 4: Coloured area of probe disappears into the pocket indicating probing depths of at least 6 mm.

Code 3: Coloured area of probe remains partly visible in the deepest pocket in the sextant.

Code 2: Coloured area of probe remains completely visible in the deepest pocket in the sextant. Supra or subgingival calculus is detected or the defective margin of a filling or crown.

Code 1: Coloured area of probe remains completely visible in the deepest pocket in the sextant. No calculus or defective margins are detected. There is bleeding after gentle probing.

Code 0: Healthy gingival tissues with no bleeding after gentle probing.

*In addition to these scores the authors recommend that the symbol * be added to the sextant score whenever there is a furcation involvement or there is total attachment loss of 7 mm or more at any site within that sextant. It should be noted that this advice differs from the BSP policy.*

The management of patients according to their sextant scores is suggested below:

Code 0: No treatment.
Code 1: Oral hygiene instruction.

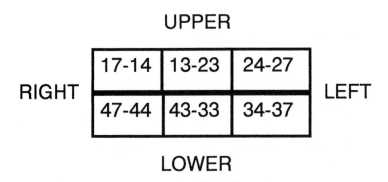

UPPER

17-14	13-23	24-27
47-44	43-33	34-37

RIGHT   LEFT

LOWER

Figure A.3 The simple system for recording the Basic Peridontal Examination (CPITH)

Code 2: OHI plus removal of calculus and correction of plaque retentive margins or fillings or crowns. Patients whose CPITN (*BPE*) score for all sextants are codes 0, 1, 2 should be screened again after an interval of 1 year.

Code 3: As code 2 but a longer time will be required for treatment. Plaque and bleeding scores are collected at the start and finish of treatment. Probing depths in the sextants scoring code 3 will be taken at the finish of treatment. Subsequently these records should be taken at intervals of not more than 1 year along with CPITN screening of other sextants.

Code 4: A full probing depth chart is required or together with recordings of gingival recession, furcation involvement and any other relevant clinical details. Individual intra-oral radiographs will be taken of teeth which show furcation involvement or loss of attachment of 7 mm or more at any site.

Code *: Treatment will include oral hygiene instruction, removal of calculus and overhangs and root planing. Re-examination is then required to assess the results of treatment to date and the need for further treatment which may include periodontal surgery.

Practitioners may wish to refer patients with scores 4 or * for specialist care.

It should be noted that this screening system is not intended to be used for monitoring purposes during treatment. Readers are referred to the BSP policy document for recording and monitoring methods suited to this purpose.

Gingival indices

Gingival indices are used to assess the level of inflammation and therefore the degree of activity of the periodontal lesions. To increase the reliability of the assessment they are always combined with other observations before making a clinical decision about the activity of the lesion.

Gingival index (Loe and Silness, 1963)

The mesial, facial, distal and lingual surface of each tooth to be assessed is examined and graded according to the following codes:

Code 0: Normal gingiva.

Code 1: Mild inflammation, slight change in colour, slight oedema, no bleeding on probing.

Code 2: Moderate inflammation, redness, oedema and glazing. Bleeding on probing.

Code 3: Severe inflammation, marked redness and oedema or ulceration. Tendency to spontaneous haemorrhage.

The codes may be totalled to give a gross score or divided by the number of points and teeth to give a mean. Alternatively, the number of readings of each code may be noted separately, to give a more statistically meaningful result.

Bleeding index (Cowell *et al.*, 1975)

Grade 0: No bleeding on gentle probing with a blunt probe.
Grade 1: Bleeding on blunt probing up to 30 s later.
Grade 2: Immediate bleeding on blunt probing.
Grade 3: Spontaneous bleeding.

Gingival bleeding index (Ainamo and Bay, 1975)

This variation of the bleeding index has the distinct advantage of using the presence or absence of bleeding as its criterion. This improves the reliability of the recording.
Code 0: No bleeding after gentle probing with a blunt probe.
Code 1: Bleeding 10 s after gentle probing with a blunt probe.

Plaque indices

Plaque indices are used to measure the amount of clinical microbial plaque on the teeth. The most used is the Plaque Index of Silness and Loe (1964) which is described below. Another useful modification of this is the modified plaque index which uses the presence or absence of clinical plaque deposits as its criterion.

Plaque index

(Silness and Loe, 1964)
Code 0: Normal gingiva.

Code 1: A film of plaque, visible only by removal on a probe or by disclosing.
Code 2: Moderate accumulations of plaque within the pockets or on the margins which can be seen with the naked eye.
Code 3: Heavy accumulations of soft material filling the niche between the gingival margin and tooth surface. The interdental area is filled with debris.

Modified plaque index

One variation of the plaque index that is often used is to record presence or absence (1 or 0), usually after staining with a disclosing agent. This method has a number of advantages, including being quicker to undertake, having less variation within and between examiners, and being easier to analyse than the multiple codes of the other indices.

Code 0: No clinical plaque deposits visible in the gingival area.
Code 1: Plaque deposits visible after disclosing in the gingival area.

Mobility index (Grace and Smales, 1989)

Grade 0: No apparent mobility.
Grade 1: Perceptible mobility but less than 1 mm buccolingually.
Grade 2: Definite mobility between 1 and 2 mm buccolingually.
Grade 3: Gross mobility exceeding 2 mm buccolingually and/or vertical mobility.

It should be noted that, in order to distinguish mobility grades from pocket depths, they are usually recorded in Roman numerals on periodontal charts, e.g. I, II, III.

Caries indices

The use of caries indices for studying disease patterns in different populations has revealed much about the nature of dental caries. The prevalence of dental caries in a population gives an indication of the number of people who are affected by the disease and the incidence indicates the rate at which it progresses. Epidemiology is the study of disease in populations rather than individuals.

It has been revealed by dental epidemiological studies that in most western countries dental caries rates in children are falling, while in Third World countries the reverse is true. This has been discovered using a measurement that reflects the extent of disease. In the case of dental caries the DMF index is used. The letters DMF stand for: D, the number of decayed teeth with carious lesions; M, teeth which have been extracted and are therefore missing; F, the number of teeth which contain restorations or fillings.

The DMF index can be further refined to indicate decayed, missing and filled teeth, DMF(T). Decayed, missing and filled surfaces, DMF(S), is a further refinement of the index for use in permanent teeth. A very similar index is used for deciduous teeth except that capital letters are not used. Here, def(t) or def(s) are used where e stands for extracted teeth rather than those exfoliated in the normal way.

The use of these indices can present a few problems because in young children teeth may have been lost due to normal exfoliation, whereas in older children teeth may have been lost due to trauma or orthodontic reasons.

In adults, tooth loss may be due to periodontal disease and not caries, so use of these indices must be clearly defined at the beginning of any study.

Selected bibliography

Ainamo, J. and Bay, I. (1975) Problems and proposals for recording plaque and gingivitis. *International Dental Journal*, **25,** 229–235.

British Society of Periodontology: Periodontology in General Dental Practice in the United Kingdom. A first policy statement. Available from The Secretary, British Society of Periodontology, Charles Clifford Dental Hospital, Sheffield S10 2SZ, United Kingdom.

Cowell, C. R., Saxton, C. A., Sheiham, A. and Wagg, B. J. (1975) Testing therapeutic measures for controlling gingivitis: procedures in man, a suggested protocol. *Journal of Clinical Periodontology*, **2,** 231–240.

Egelberg, J. (1970) A review of the development of dental plaque. In *Dental Plaque* (ed. W. D. McHugh), Livingstone, Edinburgh, pp. 9–16.

Loe, H. and Silness, J. (1963) Periodontal disease in pregnancy. I: Prevalence and severity. *Acta Odontologica Scandinavica*, **21,** 533–551.

Radiation Protection in Dental Practice: Standing Dental Advisory Committee. (1990) Department of Health, London.

Silness, J. and Loe, H. (1964) Periodontal disease in pregnancy. II: Correlation between oral hygiene and periodontal conditions. *Acta Odontologica Scandinavica*, **22,** 121–135.

Further reading

Basic dental sciences

Bercovitz, B. K. S., Holland, G. R. and Moxham, B. J. (1987) *A Colour Atlas and Textbook of Oral Anatomy*. Wolfe Medical Publications, London.

Darby, M. L. and Bushee, E. J. (1986) *Mosby's Comprehensive Review of Dental Hygiene*. C. V. Mosby, St. Louis.

Longmore, R. B. and McRae, D. A. (1985) *Clinical Anatomy for Dentistry*. Churchill Livingstone, Edinburgh.

Scully, C. and Flint, S. (1989) *An Atlas of Stomatology, Oral Disease and Manifestations of Systemic Disease*. Martin Dunitz Ltd, London.

van Beek, G. C. (1983) *Dental Morphology: An Illustrated Guide*. Wright, Bristol.

Dental deposits

ten Cate, J. M. (1989) *Recent Advances in the Study of Dental Calculus*. Oxford University Press, Oxford.

Loe, H. and Kleinman, D. V. (1986) *Dental Plaque Control Measures and Oral Hygiene Practices*. Oxford University Press, Oxford.

Patient management

Collins, W. J. N. and Walsh, T. F. (1991) *A Handbook for Dental Hygienists*, 3rd edn. Butterworth–Heinemann, Oxford.

Grace, A. M. and Smales, F. C. (1989) *Periodontal Control. An Effective System for Diagnosis, Selection, Control and Treatment Planning in General Practice*. Quintessence, London.

Locker, D. (1989) *An Introduction to Behavioural Science and Dentistry*. Routledge Publishing, London.

Manson, J. D. and Eley, B. M. (1989) *Outline of Periodontics*. Wright, Bristol.

Paul, J. E. (1980) *A Manual of Four Handed Dentistry*. Quintessence, Berlin.

Inflammatory periodontal diseases

Kieser, J. B. (1990) *Periodontics: a Practical Approach*. Wright, London.
Lindhe, J. (1989) *Textbook of Clinical Periodontology*, 2nd edn. Munksgaard, Copenhagen.
Proceedings of the World Workshop in Clinical Periodontics. The American Academy of Periodontology, 1989.

Other preventive procedures

Croser, D. and Chipping, J. (1989) *Cross Infection Control in General Dental Practice. A Practical Guide for the Whole Dental Team*. Quintessence, London.
Kidd, E. A. M. and Joyston-Bechal, S. (1987) *Essentials of Dental Caries: the Disease and its Management*. Wright, Bristol.
Mitchell, L. and Gordon, P. H. (1990) Fissure sealants – recent developments. *Dental Update*, **17**, 299–302.

Special needs

Baskar, R. M., Harrison, A. and Ralph, J. P. (1988) *Overdentures in General Dental Practice*. British Dental Association, London.
Hobkirk, J. A. (1985) *A Colour Atlas of Complete Dentures*. Wolfe Medical Publications, London.
Hunter, B. (1987) *Dental Care for Handicapped Patients. Dental Practitioner Handbook*, Wright, Bristol.

Index